Vascular Access Surgery - Tips and Tricks

Edited by Alexander E. Berezin

Published in London, United Kingdom

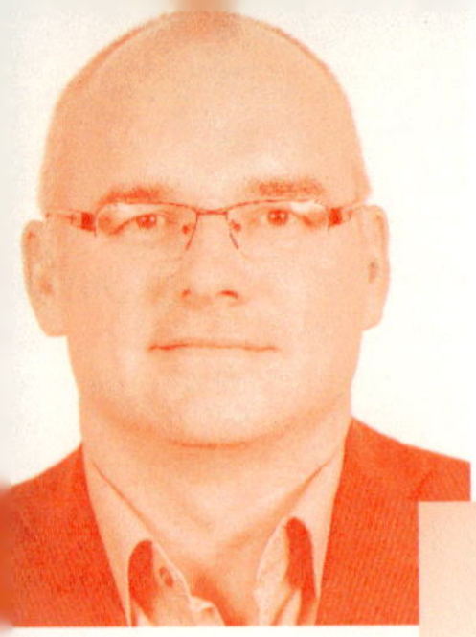
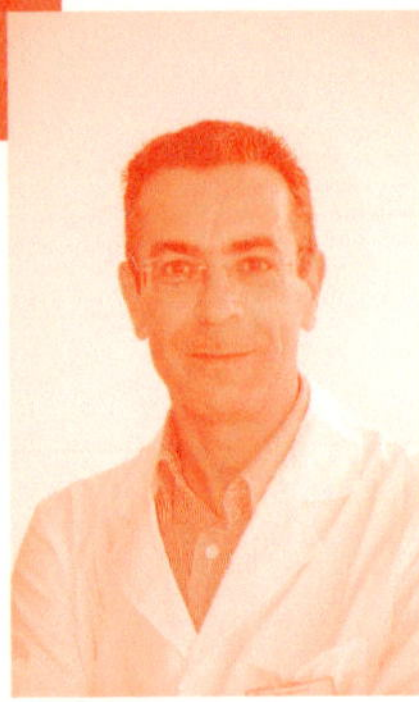
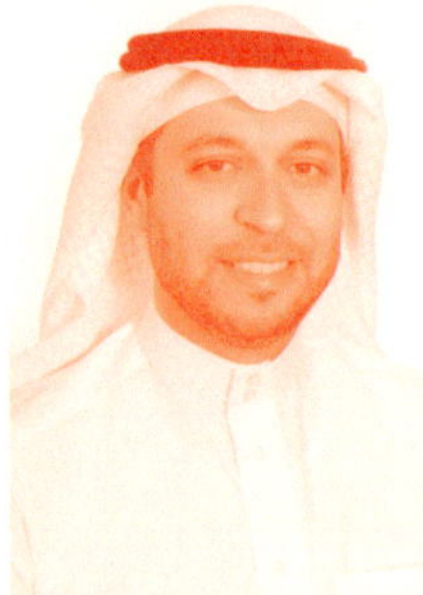
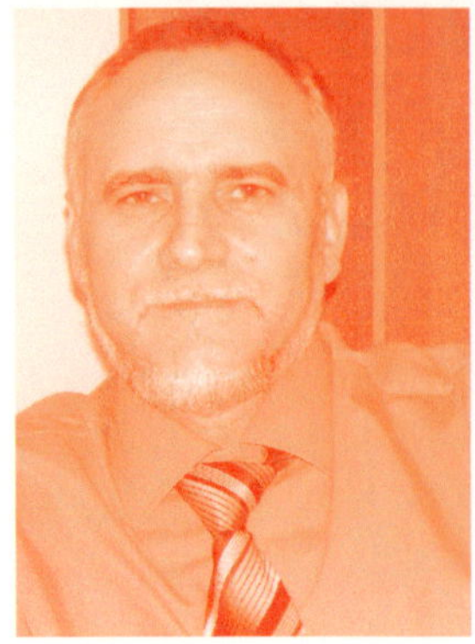
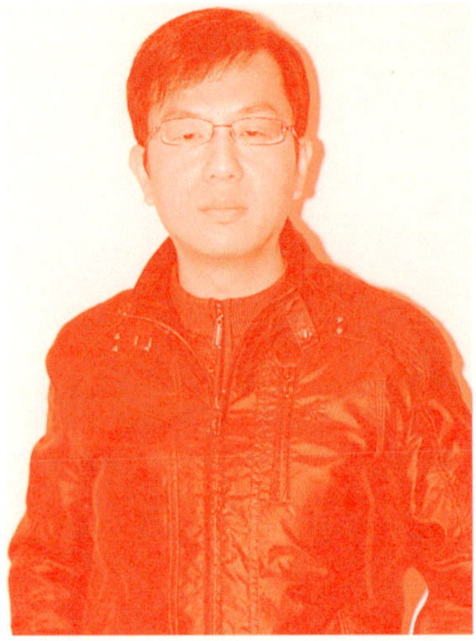
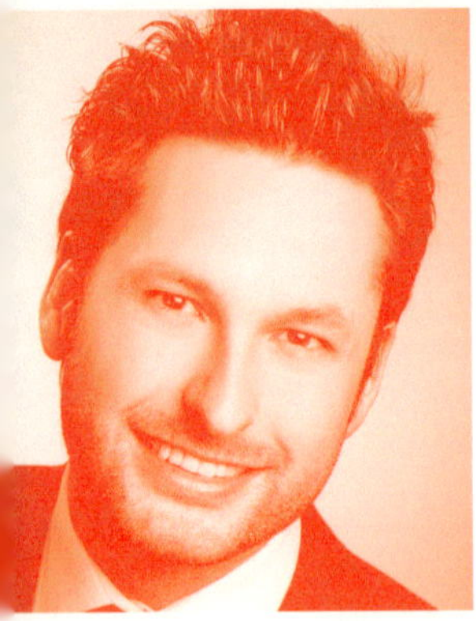
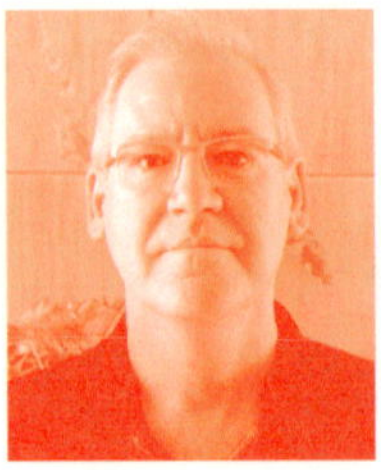

IntechOpen

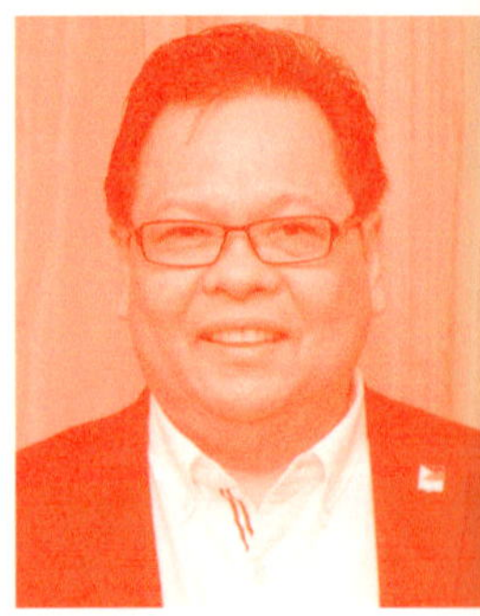
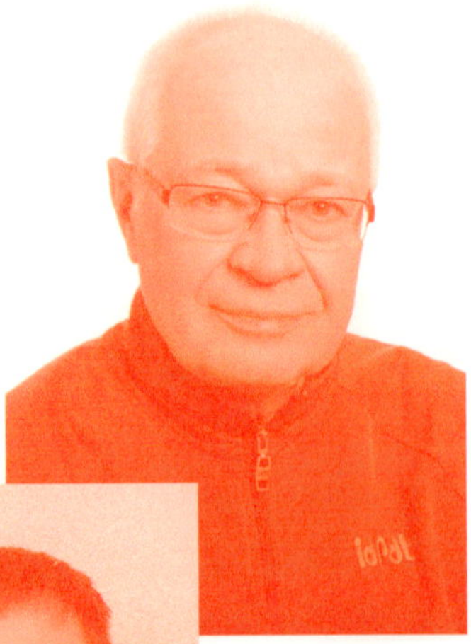
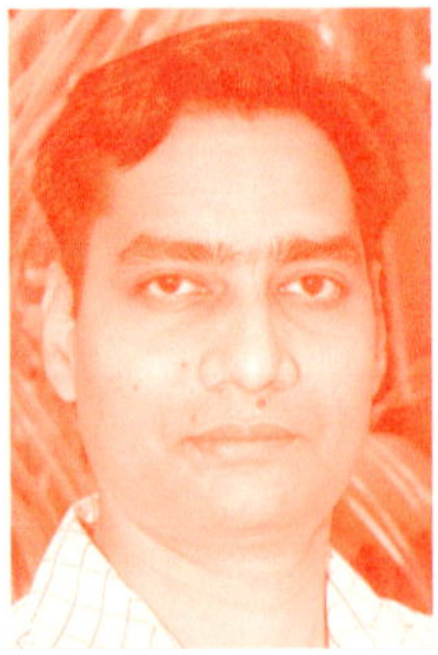
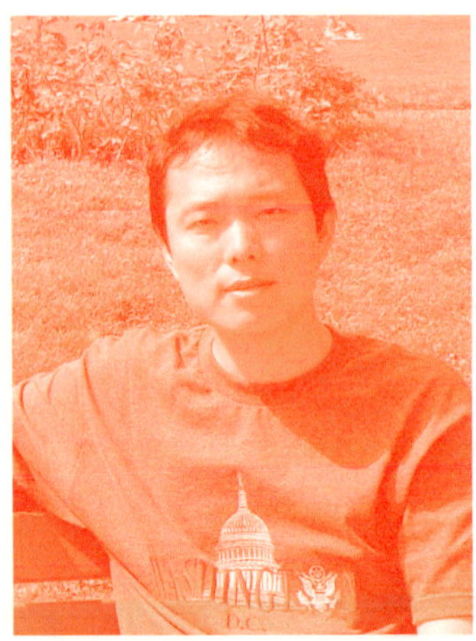
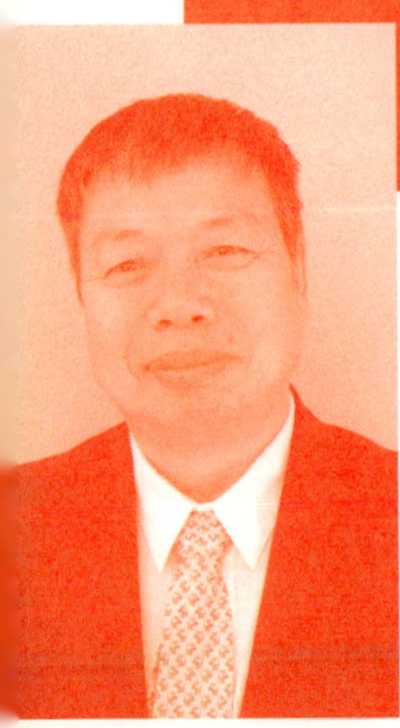
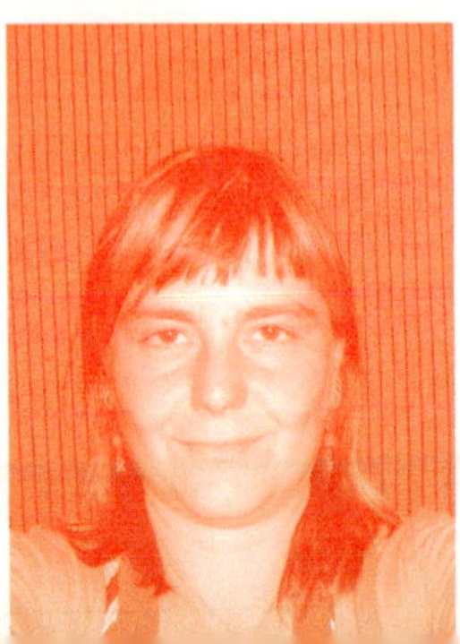

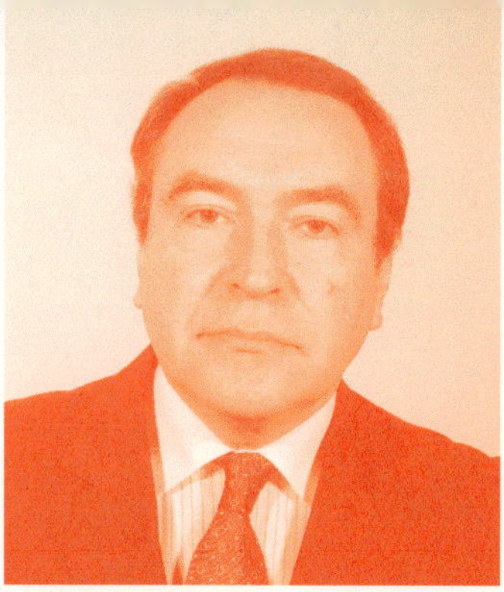

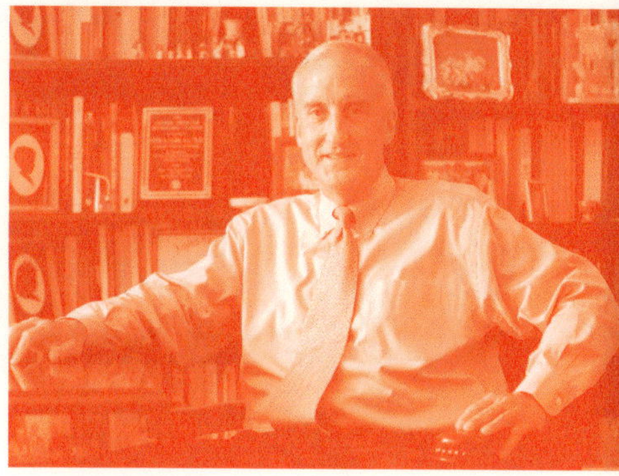

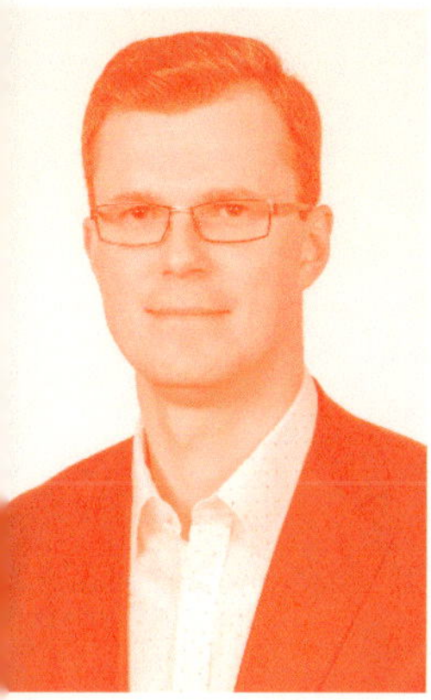

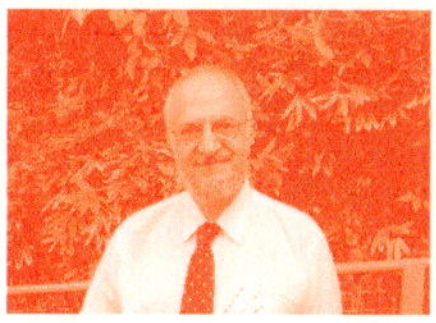

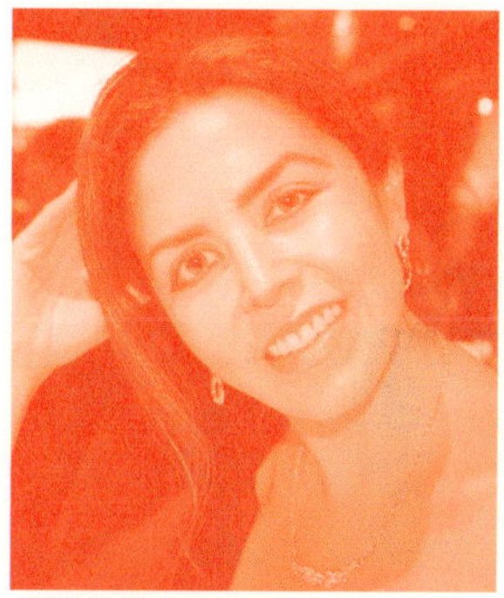

Supporting open minds since 2005

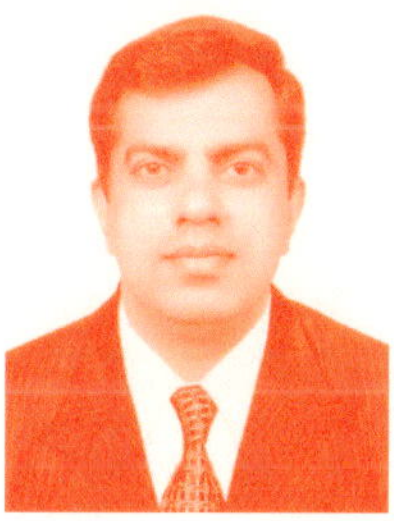

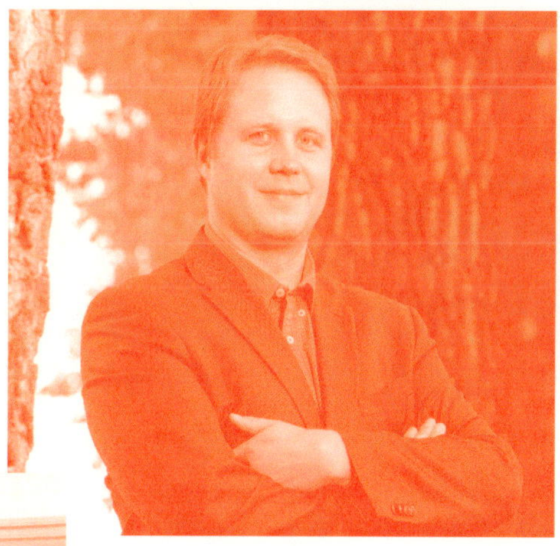

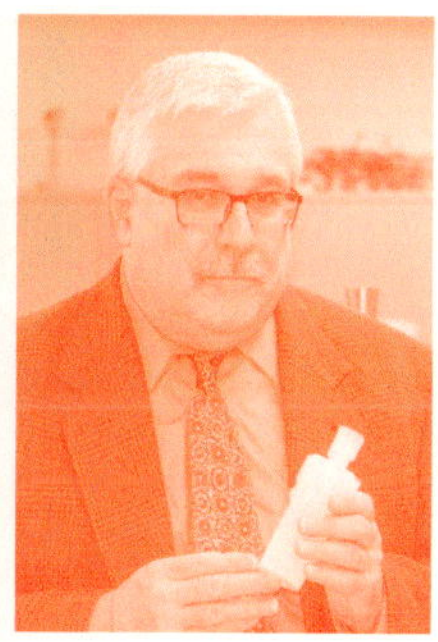

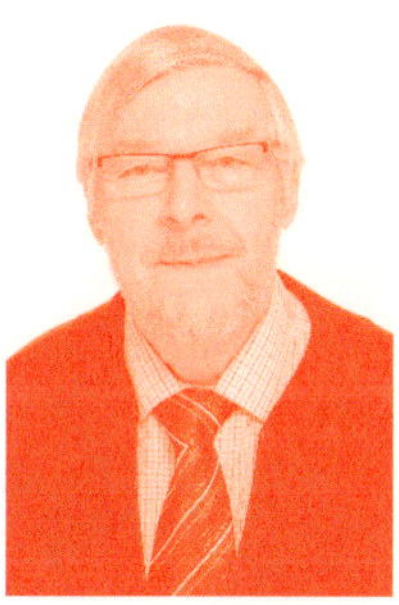

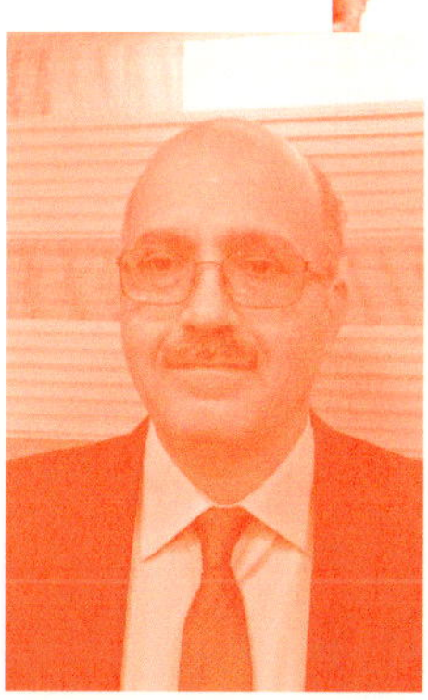

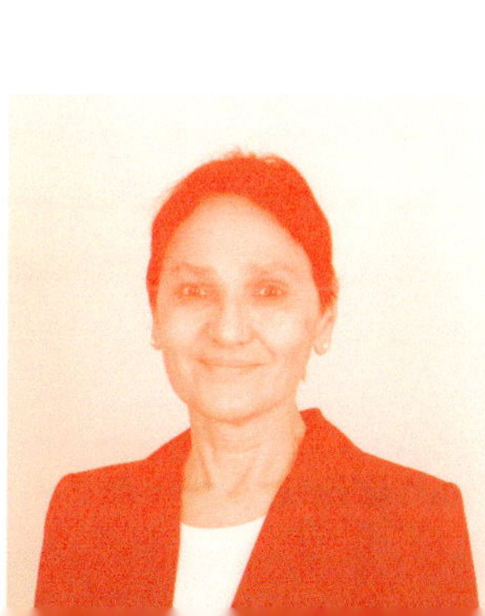

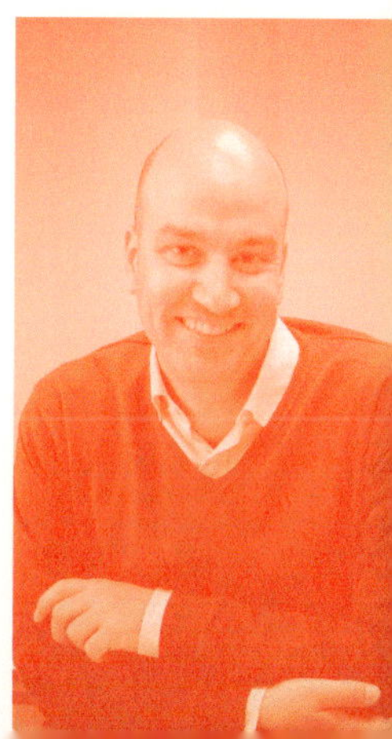

Vascular Access Surgery - Tips and Tricks
http://dx.doi.org/10.5772/intechopen.78463
Edited by Alexander E. Berezin

Contributors
David Johnson, Andrea Viecelli, Rebecca Hudson, Olga V Petyunina, Mykola Kopytsya, Iurii Rudyk, Ganna Isayeva, Kevin Dale Mangum, Naiem Nassiri, Arash Fereydooni, Mohd. Shahbaaz Khan, Joerg Rammo, Bernard Canaud, Pedro Ponce, Stefano Stuard, Maria Teresa Parisotto, Ellen Busink, Christian Apel

First published in London, United Kingdom, 2019 by IntechOpen
IntechOpen is the global imprint of INTECHOPEN LIMITED, registered in England and Wales, registration number: 11086078, The Shard, 25th floor, 32 London Bridge Street
London, SE19SG - United Kingdom
Printed in Croatia

British Library Cataloguing-in-Publication Data
A catalogue record for this book is available from the British Library

Additional hard copies can be obtained from orders@intechopen.com

Vascular Access Surgery - Tips and Tricks
Edited by Alexander E. Berezin
p. cm.
Print ISBN 978-1-83880-171-7
Online ISBN 978-1-83880-172-4

For EU product safety concerns:
IN TECH d.o.o., Prolaz Marije Krucifikse Kozulić 3, 51000 Rijeka, Croatia, info@intechopen.com or visit our website at intechopen.com.

Meet the editor

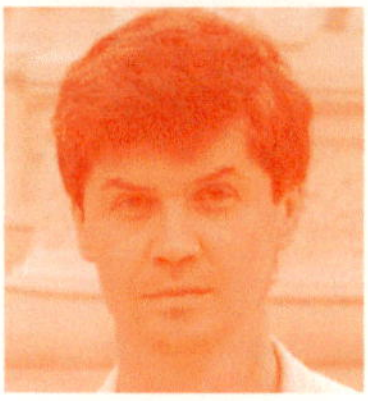

Dr. Alexander E. Berezin received his PhD in 1994 from the State Medical University of Zaporozhye (Ukraine). He is currently working as Senior Consultant, Lecturer, and Professor of the Internal Medicine Department at the same university. His research focuses on the fundamental study of developing cardiac and vascular diseases, prevention and rehabilitation, risk stratification, biological markers, and guided therapy. Based on this research and training in cardiac and vascular diseases, he has received several awards and honors. He is editor-in-chief of five highly reputed journals and has been serving as an editorial board member of scientific repute. He has published 1050 original articles/reviews in reputed journals, as well as 57 books/book chapters.

Contents

Preface

This book examines the contemporary methodology and management of vascular access for multiple purposes, including coronary intervention, dialysis, and transcatheter aortic valve implantation technology. It recognizes the impact of decision-making regarding the route of access to minimize procedural complications, especially in patients with complicated vascular anatomy. It also presents a method for regional anesthesia for vascular access surgery in the context of optimal clinical outcomes. A hybrid vascular surgery technique is also disputed. In addition, the book contains studies that address the need to reduce in-hospital clinical risk and boost long-term survival in patients who are candidates for vascular access surgery. Likewise, this book contains an assortment of discussions on the various clinical aspects of vascular access to enrich our knowledge and understanding of the contemporary methodology and management of vascular access for a broad range of purposes. The book contains four different sections: 1. Vascular Access: Methodology and Contemporary Management; 2. Vascular Access and Reparative Surgery; 3. Vascular Access Failure; and 4. Risk Stratification in Vascular Access.

Dr. Alexander E. Berezin
Professor,
Senior Consultant of the Therapeutic Unit,
Internal Medicine Department,
State Medical University of Zaporozhye, Ukraine

Section 1

Vascular Access: Methodology and Contemporary Management

Chapter 1

Different Sites of Vascular Access for Transcutaneous Aortic Valve Implantation (TAVI)

Mohd Shahbaaz Khan

Abstract

Aortic valve stenosis is a common valvular heart disease and its incidence is increasing day by day as the life expectancy is increasing gradually. It can be of congenital or acquired variety but in old ages aortic stenosis is acquired mostly and main reasons rheumatic heart disease or senile calcification of aortic valve. Aortic valve replacement with mechanical tissue valves is the surgical management of aortic valve stenosis but some of the patients are not suitable for the surgery based on their physical status and associated comorbidities. These patients are high risk for surgical complications or they have prohibitive risks for surgery. Transcutaneous aortic valve implantation is the new technique developed to implanting aortic valve mostly without opening the sternum and without using cardiopulmonary bypass machine. This procedure is mostly done via transfemoral access but in case of contraindications to use femoral artery for access some other different accesses are used to implant the aortic valve, that is, transsubclavian/transaxillary access, transapical access, transaortic access, transcarotid and transcaval accesses. In this chapter we are going to discuss all accesses in details.

Keywords: TAVI, transfemoral access, transsubclavian access, transaxillary access, transapical access, transaortic access, transcarotid and transcaval access

1. Introduction

Aortic valve is present between left ventricle and aorta. It opens during ventricular systole and closes at ventricular diastole.

Aortic stenosis (AS) represents obstruction of blood flow across the aortic valve due to congenital or acquired narrowing. Etiology can be bicuspid aortic valve, rheumatic aortic stenosis and senile aortic stenosis due to calcification of aortic valve.

It is a progressive disease that presents after a long subclinical period with symptoms of decreased exercise capacity, exertional chest pain (angina), syncope, and heart failure.

Echocardiography helps in diagnosis and grading of the aortic stenosis (**Table 1**).

Most of the patients usually undergo open surgical aortic valve replacement with mechanical or bioprosthetic aortic valve, but some patients may not be suitable

Table1-Grading of aortic stenosis			
Grade	Aortic Jet velocity (m/s)	Mean gradient (mmHg)	Valve area (cm2)
Normal	≤2	<5	3.0-4.0
Mild	≤3	<25	>1.5
Moderate	3.0-4.0	25-40	1.0-1.5
Severe	>4.0	>40	<1.0

Table 1.
Grading of aortic stenosis.

candidate for the open surgical aortic valve replacement because of their associated comorbidities or risk of adverse outcome.

Transcatheter aortic valve implantation (TAVI) is the procedure of implanting the prosthetic aortic valve through intravascular route. First transcatheter aortic valve implantation was done by Cribier et al. [1].

It is the preferred procedure for the severe aortic stenosis patients who are being considered as non-operable [2] or high risk procedure [3] for open surgical aortic valve replacement.

It has become a well-established procedure over the years and since its invention over hundreds of thousands of valves has been deployed. This number is gradually increasing day by day.

There is a basic idea of a crimped aortic bioprosthetic valve and its transcatheter implantation in aortic valve position.

Followings (**Table 2**) are the aspects to be considered by the heart team to take decision for management of severe aortic stenosis in high risk patients for surgical aortic valve replacement or TAVI.

There are many ways of implanting the aortic valve (**Figure 1**) by TAVI but most commonly used route is retrograde transfemoral arterial access. This is less invasive and the only percutaneous way of implanting the aortic valve. Even it can be done without general anesthesia. Other routes need surgical cut down for the arterial access.

Peripheral vessels must be assessed for the size, tortuosity, and calcification of the iliac and femoral arteries. Vascular assessment is most commonly performed using contrast angiography or CT angiography. By default transfemoral access is considered to be vascular access site for TAVI.

Other retrograde transcatheter aortic valve implantation (TAVI) is currently performed through an alternative access in 15% of patients. Existing data does not favor one route over another one. All the routes have different advantages and disadvantages.

This chapter will review the different accesses for aortic valve implantation.

Most common vascular access for TAVI is transfemoral artery by default. As the technology has improved, the options for the vascular access for TAVI has increased and may include transfemoral, transsubclavian (transaxillary), transapical, trans-aortic, and transcaval.

With the availability of the lower profile aortic valves for implantation, these valves are mostly deployed via transfemoral route but in case of contra-indication to use femoral artery for TAVI other vessels are used for access; as in case femoral arteries are of small size, tortuous or heavily calcified.

Before proceeding for TAVI, patient should undergo full work up with coronary angiography, CT angiography scan of heart, aorta and peripheral vessels, transthoracic and transesophageal echocardiography, lab investigations and other radiological investigations.

	Favors TAVI	Favors SAVR
Clinical Characteristics		
STS/Euro SCORE II <4% (Logistic Euro SCORE I <10%)		+
STS/Euro SCORE II ≥4% (Logistic Euro SCORE I ≥10%)	+	
Presence of severe comorbidity (not adequately reflected by scores)	+	
Age <75 years		+
Age ≥75 years	+	
Previous cardiac surgery	+	
Frailty	+	
Restricted mobility and conditions that may affect the rehabilitation process after the procedure	+	
Suspicion of endocarditis		+
Anatomical and technical aspect		
Favorable access for trans femoral TAVI	+	
Unfavorable access(any) for TAVI		+
Sequelae of chest radiation	+	
Porcelain aorta	+	
Presence of intact coronary artery bypass grafts at risk when sternotomy is performed	+	
Expected patient-prosthesis mismatch	+	
Severe chest deformation or scoliosis	+	
Short distance between coronary Ostia and aortic valve annulus		+
Size of aortic valve annulus out of range for TAVI		+
Aortic root morphology unfavorable for TAVI		+
Valve morphology (bicuspid, degree of calcification, calcification pattern) unfavorable for TAVI		+
Presence of thrombi in aorta or LV		+
Cardiac condition in addition to aortic stenosis that require consideration for concomitant intervention		
Severe CAD require revascularization with CABG		+
Severe primary mitral valve disease, which could be treated surgically		+
Severe tricuspid valve disease		+
Aneurysm of ascending aorta		+
Sepal hypertrophy requiring myectomy		+

Table 2.
Factors to be considered in severe Aortic stenosis in high risk patients for Surgical AVR or TAVI.

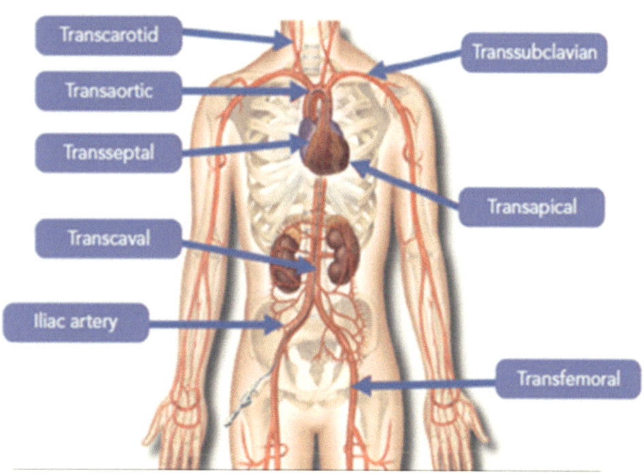

Figure 1.
Different routes of aortic valve implantation by TAVI.

Although in most of the TAVI procedures, Cardiopulmonary bypass (CPB) is not required but patient should have a full informed consent with possibility of emergency midline sternotomy and use of CPB in case of complications.

While it is difficult to predict which patients will need temporary CPB support during or after valve deployment, usually patients with ejection fraction (<25%) with severe pulmonary hypertension, especially those requiring significant inotropes during and after anesthetic induction are at higher risk.

2. Preoperative assessment and planning

Potential TAVI patients must undergo full evaluation with

- Coronary angiography
- Transthoracic echocardiography (TTE)
- Transesophageal echocardiography (TEE)
- Cardiac computed tomography
- CT angiography of aorta and peripheral vessels

Initial TAVI evaluation should include an assessment of the following variables also:

1. Severity of aortic stenosis.
2. Anatomy of the aortic valve.
3. Aortic valve calcification.
4. Annular, sinotubular, and sinus of Valsalva dimensions.
5. Ventricular function.
6. Coronary artery disease.
7. Height of coronary ostia from aortic annulus.
8. Ileofemoral vessel size, calcification, and tortuosity.

Patients with severe coronary artery disease and lesions which are treatable by percutaneous coronary intervention should get stents prior to the procedure. We keep patients on dual anti platelets therapy for about 6 weeks and then take them for TAVI.

The aortic annulus is sized at mid-systole, and the valve size is selected based upon 10% over-sizing of the annular diameter.

If the annulus is not adequately sized, there would be risk of improper valve size selection that could lead to paravalvular leak, valve embolization, coronary obstruction if the sinus of Valsalva is small or the distance between the annulus and the coronary ostia is less (<10 mm).

DOI: http://dx.doi.org/10.5772/intechopen.84533

3. Transfemoral access

3.1 Introduction

Transfemoral access (**Figure 2**) is the most preferred route in majority of the TAVI procedures world over [4] unless there is an increased risk of vascular complications depending on vascular size, tortuosity and calcification [5].

3.2 Planning

- All patients should undergo a CT-angiographic scan with 3D reconstruction of aorta and femoral vessels
- Aorta should be assessed for tortuosity, presence of aneurysms, atherosclerotic plaques and aortic arch calcifications
- Minimum size of femoral and iliac arteries should be more than 5.5 mm (ideally more than 6.5 mm) and it should be free of calcification
- A circumferential calcification could be a potential contraindication for transfemoral approach
- Some studies shown that a sheath to femoral artery ratio of greater than 1.05 is predictive of a vascular complication [6]
- Bifurcation of femoral artery and its relation with the femoral head should be evaluated properly
- Site of needle entry may be altered based on CT scan or ultrasound findings of high bifurcation of the common femoral artery and presence of significant calcium.

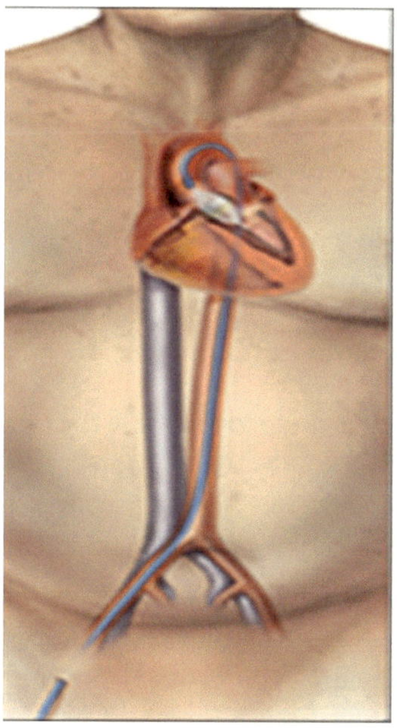

Figure 2.
Transfemoral access for TAVI.

3.3 Technique

- Patient lies supine on operating table
- Endotracheal intubation, arterial line and central line with temporary pace maker lead through right internal jugular vein and placed
- Surgical part painted and draped from neck down till mid-thigh
- Femoral arteries are accessed percutaneously under vascular ultrasound or fluoroscopic guidance
- Surgical cut down can be considered in obese patients with deep femoral arteries
- 6Fr sheath is inserted in one femoral artery and then a 5 Fr pigtail catheter is placed in non-coronary sinus of aorta as a marker for aortic valve placement and positioning.
- These days routinely we are using right radial artery for placing Pigtail catheter in non-coronary sinus of aorta instead of femoral artery
- IV heparin is given to keep activated clotting time (ACT) around 200–250 s.
- Another femoral artery is used to insert 18 Fr valve deployment sheath. First a 6 Fr sheath is inserted and then a soft, J-tipped wire is placed into the descending thoracic aorta (DTA).
- Two percutaneous sutures based vascular closure devices (Per close devices) are placed, which are used to control the bleeding after the procedure.
- The soft J-tipped wire and an exchange catheter are inserted into the aorta
- A soft wire is exchanged for a super-stiff Amplatz wire
- Then catheter and 6-Fr sheath are removed
- 18 Fr sheath is inserted after making a small nick with 11 blade at the puncture site in order to facilitate entry of bigger sheath
- Valve deployment is done through the 18-Fr sheath
- Contra lateral pigtail catheter should be pulled out a little before the opening the valve fully; to prevent the entrapment of the pigtail catheter in device
- Rapid ventricular pacing is done to decrease the blood pressure and valve is deployed under fluoroscopic and transesophageal echocardiographic guidance
- At completion of the procedure we reverse the ACT by giving protamine and then remove the deployment sheath first and control bleeding by per close devices.
- In case of doubtful control of bleeding or suspicion of femoral artery stenosis, we do check angiography using cross over from the contralateral femoral artery
- We usually extubate the patient in operating room

4. Transsubclavian/axillary access

4.1 Introduction

The subclavian artery has recently become a site of access for TAVI [7]. Right axillary or subclavian artery is rarely used for TAVI because of anatomic restrictions and unfavourable angle for valve implantation. The proximal third of the left axillary artery (between the lateral border of the first rib and the medial border of the pectoralis minor) represents the ideal target for both surgical and percutaneous approaches.

A study suggested that subclavian access is not advisable in patients with subclavian artery diameter <7 mm, significant tortuosity, or prior coronary artery bypass grafting (CABG) and patent in situ internal mammary artery grafts [8].

4.2 Disadvantages

There is a higher risk of stroke due to interruption of blood flow to the vertebral arteries in patients with carotid disease who depend on the vertebral arteries for cerebral perfusion.

4.3 Planning

- CT angio scan with 3D reconstruction of the subclavian and axillary arteries.
- Vessel size should be >6.5 mm without calcifications and tortuosity
- It is more prone for vascular complications (especially in old age) because of anatomical differences between subclavian/axillary (more elastic fibers and less muscular wall) and femoral arteries.
- Post CABG patients in whom LIMA was used for LAD anastomosis, this approach can be lethal due to acute graft occlusion.

4.4 Technique

- A femoral artery and vein access is obtained, 6 Fr sheath is inserted and then pigtail catheter is placed in the aortic sinus and a femoral transvenous temporary pacing lead inserted through femoral vein.
- Surgical cutdown for the left axillary artery is done in deltopectoral groove (6–7 cm in size and 1 cm below and parallel to the clavicle from the mid clavicular line to the axillary line) (**Figure 3**)
- Axillary artery is exposed by dissection of pectoralis major and lateral retraction of the pectoralis minor
- Purse string suture is placed on the artery
- The patient is heparinized to maintain an ACT 200–250 s
- A sheath is inserted by direct puncture Using the Seldinger technique

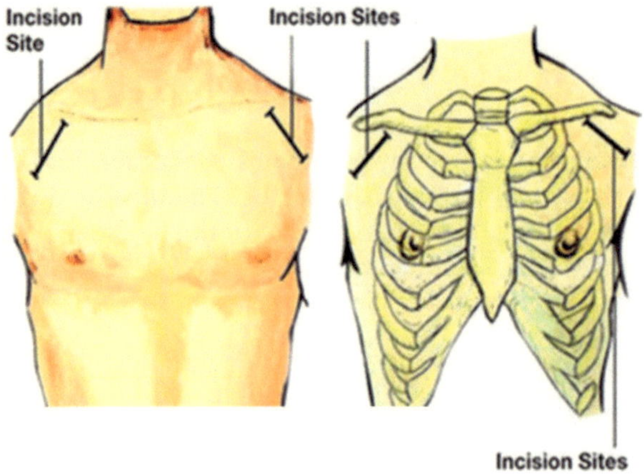

Figure 3.
Transsubclavian artery access.

- In some selected cases an 8–10 mm sized Dacron graft can be anastomosed in an end-to-side fashion and then cannulated with the valve deployment sheath
- A fully percutaneuos approach was described in 2012 as the "*Hamburg Sankt George Approach*" [9]
- Once the sheath is in place, aortic valve is deployed in same manner as for previously described transfemoral access
- Heparin reversal, sheath removal and control of vascular bleeding are done in same way as transfemoral approach.

5. Transapical access

5.1 Introduction

Transapical access (**Figure 4**) is the alternative approach for TAVI in patients in whom transfemoral or transsubclavian/transaxillary approach is not feasible.

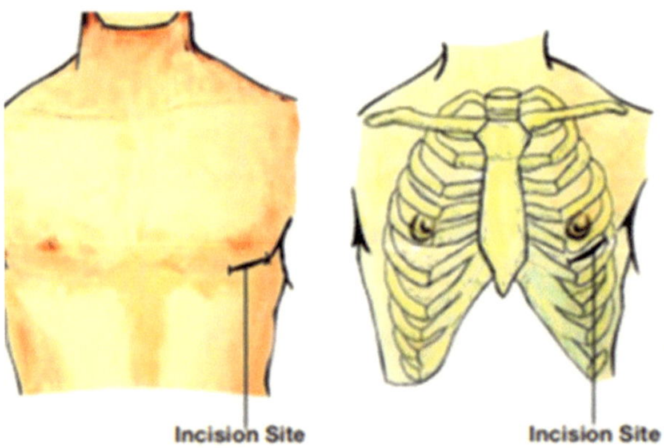

Figure 4.
Transapical access for TAVI.

5.2 Advantages

The transapical approach has the following advantages over other approaches:

1. Peripheral vascular anatomy and size are not limitation

2. The valve is easily crossed in the antegrade direction (vs. retrograde)

3. Less paravalvular leaks

4. Shorter time for insertion and lesser contrast use

5.3 Disadvantages

1. Longer recovery due to thoracotomy

2. Bleeding

3. Not suitable for patients with significant lung disease (forced expiratory volume in 1 s <35%) or low ejection fraction (<15–20%) [10]

4. It could be a source of postoperative Left ventricular (LV) pseudoaneurysm, and may impair left ventricular function

5.4 Planning

- Preoperative CT scan chest is needed to identify both the rib space over the apex of the heart and the distance from the sternum to the LV apex

- CPB should be standby, to use in case of emergent conversion to open AVR

- Cannulation sites for CPB must be planned

- Common femoral artery and vein are used for cannulation usually

- Access to femoral vessels must be done in beginning of case, if femoral vessels are supposed to be used as a bailout CPB cannulation (on the contra lateral side, other than from the femoral arterial access for pigtail aortogram and venous access for ventricular pacing

- Axillary artery can also be cannulated in case femoral artery is small in size

- A final bailout for CPB is transapical cannulation itself putting a long arterial cannula across the aortic valve. The obvious advantage of this approach is that area will already be readily accessible. The disadvantage of the transapical CPB cannulation is that it gives up the site of access for valve deployment

- It need to be careful while tying the sutures as LV can tear due to friable myocardium

5.5 Technique

- It is done under general anesthesia

- The procedure should be performed in a hybrid operative room

- Supine position with both arms tucked at the sides and a small roll under the left chest
- It is important to prep patient widely to include all potential CPB cannulation sites and for an antero lateral thoracotomy
- Femoral artery and vein access is achieved as routinely
- A femoral transvenous pacing lead is inserted in right ventricle and a pigtail catheter is placed in aortic root via femoral artery
- Anterolateral thoracotomy is made in the fifth or sixth intercostal space
- Dissection is carried down to the pleura and a rib retractor is placed
- After identifying the phrenic nerve, the pericardium is opened
- In cases of a previous sternotomy, adhesions are released between the pericardium and epicardium for adequate exposure of the LV apex
- Two apical concentric pledgeted 3–0 PROLENE purse-string sutures are placed just cephalad to the apex and lateral to the LAD coronary artery
- The purse-string sutures must be deep into the myocardium as they are prone to tear through the ventricular tissue.
- The patient is heparinized to maintain an ACT 200–250 s
- Fluoroscopy is used to align all three aortic cusps in the same plane asin transfemoral approach
- The Left ventricle is punctured with a needle and a 0.035″ J wire is passed into the LV, across the aortic valve and into the ascending aorta
- The needle is exchanged for a 7-French sheath
- The 0.035″ guide wire is then exchanged for an Amplatz super-stiff wire
- The 7-French sheath is exchanged for the appropriate transapical delivery sheath
- If there is bleeding around the sheath, the purse-string sutures can be snared
- The bioprosthetic valve is delivered through the sheath and positioned across the aortic valve
- The valve is aligned parallel to the long axis of the aorta and perpendicular to the aortic annulus [11]
- Both transesophageal echocardiography (TEE) and aortic root angiogram under fluoroscopy are used to confirm the position of the valve

- Once the optimal position is confirmed, the valve is deployed during rapid ventricular pacing
- The valve delivery apparatus is then removed leaving the stiff wire across the bioprosthesis
- TEE and angiography are used to assess valve position and paravalvular leak
- Balloon dilation may be performed if there is ≥2+ paravalvular leak
- Once satisfactory valve function and position is confirmed, all catheters and wires are removed from the apex, and purse-string sutures are tightened during rapid ventricular pacing
- Protamine is given, and additional pledgeted sutures may be placed for adequate hemostasis
- The pericardium can be closed partially and a flexible Blake drain is placed in the left pleural space with part of it in the pericardium as well for the drainage
- Thoracotomy wound is closed in layers.

6. Transaortic access

6.1 Introduction

The transaortic approach was originally reported by Bapat et al. [12, 13]. The concept behind this first report was the use of the short transapical TAVI delivery system for the retrograde TAVI implant through the ascending aorta. Since then it has become a valid option in case of severe peripheral vascular disease [14].

6.2 Advantages

It has many practical advantages compared to other approaches:

1. It avoids thoracotomy which could potentially impedes pulmonary function in COPD patients
2. It avoids cannulation of the left ventricular apex
3. It is easier to achieve hemostasis in aorta than in LV due to fragile myocardium
4. If needed, direct visualization of the aorta permits rapid cannulation and initiation of cardiopulmonary bypass for support

6.3 Disadvantages

1. It is technically challenging in case of previous sternotomy and internal mammary artery or saphenous vein grafts for CABG
2. It cannot be used in patients with porcelain aorta [15]

6.4 Planning

- Preoperative CT scan is done to shows the relationship of the distal ascending aorta to the sternum, calcification, and the distance from the distal aortic cannulation site to the aortic root
- This distance should be ideally >7 cm allowing enough space for the valve implantation.
- CPB should be standby for any intra operative complication

6.5 Technique

- It needs a hybrid operating room where fluoroscopy and TEE
- Supine position with the lower neck remaining exposed for a counter incision for the delivery sheath
- Femoral arterial access is obtained as routine for placing a pigtail catheter in the aortic sinus
- A femoral transvenous pacing lead is placed in the right ventricle
- It can be performed by two approaches. The first is through mini-sternotomy (**Figure 5**) and the second is by a right mini-thoracotomy (**Figure 6**).
- An upper ministernotomy is performed with extension to the second intercostal space, where the "J" is completed
- The pericardium is opened
- Pericardial stay sutures are placed for retraction. The aorta is then inspected to find a suitable place for catheter insertion
- It should be free from calcification and at least 6–8 cm from the aortic valve for valve deployment
- Two aortic purse strings are placed

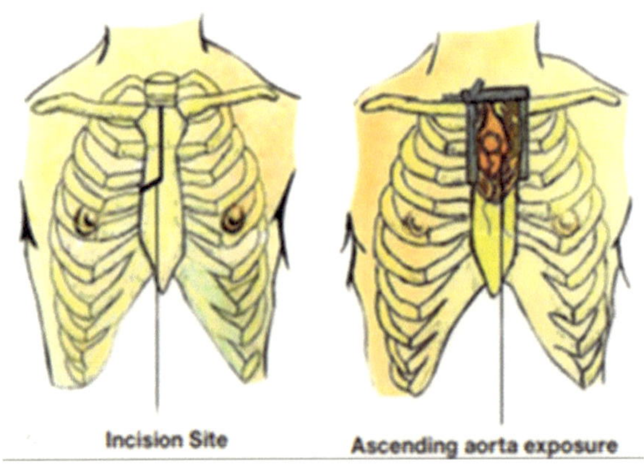

Figure 5.
Transaortic access by upper "J" ministernotomy forTAVI.

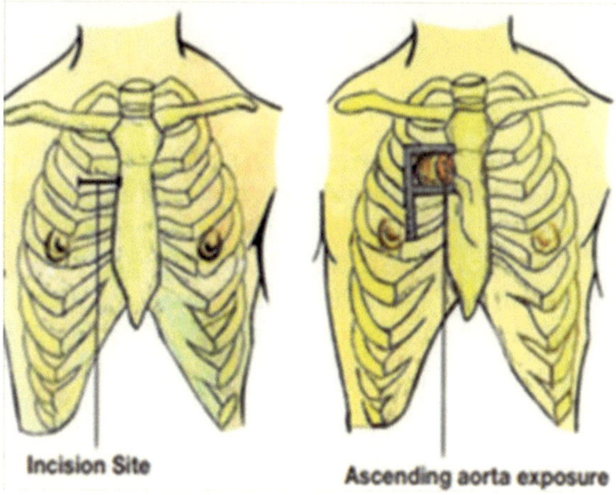

Figure 6.
Transaortic right anterior minithoracotomy for TAVI.

- The patient is heparinized to maintain an ACT 200–250 s
- An 18-gauge needle with a 0.035″ soft J guide wire is passed through the counter incision in the lower neck and used to puncture the aorta through the purse strings
- The needle is exchanged for a 7-F sheath, and a multipurpose catheter with a straight soft wire is used to cross the valve
- This is exchanged for a 0.035″ Amplatz extra-stiff J wire
- The appropriate valve sheath is placed 2–4 cm into the aorta
- An aortic root aortogram is performed to align all the three leaflets of the aortic valve in same plane
- The valve is placed through the delivery sheath and positioned across the valve
- Once optimal positioning of the valve is confirmed, rapid ventricular pacing at 160–200 beats/min is started
- When the valve is positioned correctly, the valve is deployed
- Aortograms and TEE is used to assess position and presence of any paravalvular leaks and patency of coronary ostia
- After full assessment, all catheters and wires are removed and the aortic sutures are tightened
- Protamine is administered
- A small flexible chest tube is placed in the mediastinum
- Sternum is closed with stainless steel wires
- A right mini-thoracotomy (through second intercostal space) is an option if a surgeon wants to avoid sternotomy or improve visualization in the case of a horizontal or a right-sided aorta

7. Transcarotid approach

7.1 Introduction

This approach is used rarely and required in only for the patients who have contraindications to all other accesses. Modine reported a successful series of 12 patients who underwent CoreValve TAVI with no access site complications, no stroke, and only 1 TIA contralateral to the accessed side [16].

Mylotte et al. [17] reported the feasibility and the safety of this transcarotid approach in 96 patients enrolled in 3 different French sites. In their series, no major bleedings nor vascular complications related to the access site occurred, while only three transient ischemic attacks and no strokes were reported.

7.2 Planning

- Common carotid artery diameter must be >8 mm without any calcification, stenosis or tortuosity
- CT angio carotid and brain to rule out significant atherosclerotic disease and to assess patency of the circle of Willis and cerebral circulation
- MRI brain is done assess the patency of circle of Willis.

7.3 Technique

- A 6-F sheath is placed in the femoral artery and an angled pigtail catheter is utilized for ascending aortography
- A transvenous pacing lead is placed via the femoral vein
- The right common carotid artery is exposed by vertical lower neck incision
- After proximal cross-clamping of the common carotid artery, it is opened longitudinally for 2.5 cm
- The de-aired bypass shunt is placed through the arteriotomy into the distal carotid to maintain cerebral perfusion
- Cerebral oximetry is monitored for both the cerebral hemispheres during the whole procedure
- Through the proximal portion of the arteriotomy, a 0.035-inch J-tipped wire and 7-F introducer are placed in the ascending aorta
- A multipurpose catheter is then inserted and a straight wire is used to cross the aortic valve
- The straight wire is exchanged for an Amplatz extra-stiff wire
- Under TEE and fluoroscopic guidance bioprosthetic valve is deployed as in other approaches
- After the procedure the wires, catheters, and sheath are removed, and the carotid artery is repaired with a pericardial patch.

8. Transcaval approach

8.1 Introduction

The transcaval approach, described by Greenbaum et al. [18] is considered as the last resort in patients not qualifying for any other vascular access. In the transcaval approach (**Figure 7**), the delivery system is inserted through the femoral vein and crossed to the arterial system by creating an aortocaval fistula, which is closed with an Amplatzer device after the valve is deployed.

A case series demonstrated the feasibility of the transcaval TAVI, revealing a successful valve deployment in 17 of 19 patients despite a 79% rate of transfusion and a 33% rate of vascular complications [18].

8.2 Planning

The location of the fistula is determined by a careful evaluation of the CT abdomen and pelvis prior to the procedure.

8.3 Technique

- A baseline CT-scan to identify a calcium free target on the right abdominal aortic wall allowing for a safe passage from the inferior vena cava to the aortic lumen of the large bore sheath

- After having obtained a femoral venous access, the inferior vena cava is punctured by means of a stiff CTO wire mounted over a microcatheter and a standard RCA or IMA guiding catheter

- The caval and aortic walls are perforated by using electrocautery applied at the distal end of the wire.

- Once the access is obtained to the aortic lumen, the wire is snared and both the microcatheter and the guiding catether are advanced into the abdominal aorta.

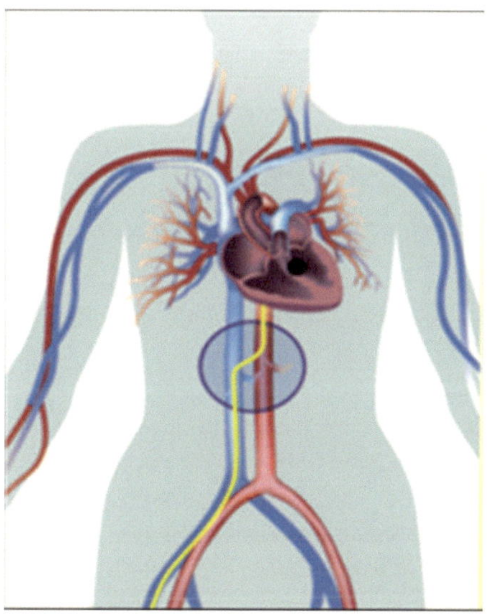

Figure 7.
Transcaval access for TAVI.

- This allows for the placement of a stiff "0.035" wire and the advancement of a large introducer sheath from the femoral vein into the aortic lumen for conventional retrograde aortic valve replacement

- At case completion, heparin is reversed, and the aortic perforation is closed using a conventional vascular, duct or ventricular septal defect occluder device.

Author details

Mohd Shahbaaz Khan
Cardio-vascular and thoracic surgeon, King Fahad Medical City, Riyadh, Kingdom of Saudi Arabia

*Address all correspondence to: mohdshahbaazkhan@yahoo.com

References

[1] Cribier A, Eltchaninoff H, Bash A, et al. Percutaneous transcatheter implantation of an aortic valve prosthesis for calcific aortic stenosis: First human case description. Circulation. 2002;**106**:3006-3008

[2] Smith CR, Leon MB, Mack MJ, et al. Transcatheter versus surgical aortic-valve replacement in high-risk patients. New England Journal of Medicine. 2011;**364**:2184-2198

[3] Leon MB, Smith CR, Mack M, et al. Transcatheter aorticvalve implantation for aortic stenosis in patients who cannot undergo surgery. The New England Journal of Medicine. 2010;**363**:1597-1607

[4] Webb JG, Chandavimol M, Thompson CR, et al. Percutaneous aortic valve implantation retrograde from the femoral artery. Circulation. 2006;**113**:842-850

[5] Schofer J, Colombo A, Klugmann S, Fajadet J, DeMarco F, Tchetche D, et al. Prospective multicenter evaluation of the direct flow medical transcatheter aortic valve. Journal of the American College of Cardiology. 2014;**63**(8):763-768

[6] Hayashida K, Lefevre T, Chevalier B, et al. Transfemoral aortic valve implantation new criteria to predict vascular complications. JACC: Cardiovascular Interventions. 2011;**4**:851-858

[7] Petronio AS, De Carlo M, Bedogni F, Marzocchi A, Klugmann S Maisano F, et al. Safety and efficacy of the subclavian approach for transcatheter aortic valve implantation with the corevalve revalving system. Circulation. Cardiovascular Interventions. 2010;**3**(4):359-366

[8] Caceres M, Braud R, Roselli EE. The axillary/subclavian artery access route for transcatheter aortic valve replacement: A systematic review of the literature. The Annals of Thoracic Surgery. 2012;**93**:1013-1018

[9] Schäfer U, Ho Y, Frerker C, Schewel D, Sanchez-Quintana D, Schofer J, et al. Direct percutaneous access technique for transaxillary transcatheter aortic valve implantation: The Hamburg Sankt Georg approach. JACC: Cardiovascular Interventions. 2012;**5**:477-486. DOI: 10.1016/j.jcin.2011.11.014

[10] Thourani VH, Gunter RL, Neravetla S, et al. Use of transaortic, transapical, and transcarotid transcatheter aortic valve replacement in inoperable patients. The Annals of Thoracic Surgery. 2013;**96**:1349-1357

[11] Walther T, Dewey T, Borger MA, et al. Transapical aortic valve implantation: Step by step. The Annals of Thoracic Surgery. 2009;**87**:276-283

[12] Bapat V, Khawaja MZ, Attia R, Narayana A, Wilson K, Macgillivray K, et al. Transaortic transcatheter aortic valve implantation using Edwards SAPIEN valve: A novel approach. Catheterization and Cardiovascular Interventions. 2012;**79**:733-740. DOI: 10.1002/ccd.23276

[13] Bapat V, Attia R. Transaortic transcatheter aortic valve implantation: Step-by-step guide. Seminars in Thoracic and Cardiovascular Surgery. 2012;**24**:206-211. DOI: 10.1053/j.semtcvs.2012.06.004

[14] Arai T, Romano M, Lefèvre T, Hovasse T, Farge A, Le Houerou D, et al. Direct comparison of feasibility and safety of transfemoral versus transaortic versus transapical transcatheter aortic valve replacement. JACC: Cardiovascular Interventions. 2016;**9**:2320-2325. DOI: 10.1016/j.jcin.2016.08.009

[15] Russo M, Tartara P. Trans-aortic transcatheter aortic valve replacement with edwards Sapien-Ascendra 3. The Cardiothoracic Surgery Network. 2014. Available from: http://www.ctsnet.org/print/ article/trans-aortic-transcatheter-aortic-valve-replacement-edwards-sapien-ascendra-3 [Accessed: 14 July, 2014]

[16] Modine T, Sudre A, Delhaye C, et al. Transcutaneous aortic valve implantation using the left carotid access: Feasibility and early clinical outcomes. The Annals of Thoracic Surgery. 2012;**93**:1489-1494

[17] Mylotte D, Sudre A, Teiger E, Obadia JF, Lee M, Spence M, et al. Transcarotid transcatheter aortic valve replacement: Feasibility and safety. JACC: Cardiovascular Interventions. 2016;**9**:472-480

[18] Greenbaum AB et al. Caval-aortic access to allow transcatheter aortic valve replacement in otherwise ineligible patients: Initial human experience. Journal of the American College of Cardiology. 2014;**63**(25 Pt A):2795-2804

Chapter 2

Vascular Access Management for Haemodialysis: A Value-Based Approach from NephroCare Experience

Bernard Canaud, Pedro Ponce, Maria Teresa Parisotto, Ellen Busink, Christian Apel, Jörg Rammo and Stefano Stuard

Abstract

A good functioning vascular access (VA) is a prerequisite to obtain a successful dialysis treatment. This chapter reviews VA management in advanced chronic kidney disease (CKD) patients drawn from the experience of a large network dialysis care provider with the following sections: overview on VA management in advanced CKD that follows patient pathway and patient profile, current practice patterns in line with best clinical practices; VA creation addressing crucial themes: when and what type of VA to construct, how to assess patient pre-emptively, how to proceed for the construction and monitoring to prevent early failures and complications; VA management with particular focus on clinical monitoring, surveillance and interventional procedures required to preserve patency and functionality of VA; the often-forgotten patient perspective is VA usage. What information to share, how to proceed for preventing pain, and fears related with VA needling? What should patients know about their VA and how to manage in daily life? Competences, skills and responsibilities of nursing staff when using and managing VA; and future of VA in terms of innovative concept for creating and maintaining VA conduits in dialysis patients.

Keywords: haemodialysis, vascular access, vascular access centre, arteriovenous fistula, arteriovenous graft, central venous catheter, vascular access complications, best nursing practice, value-based haemodialysis

1. Background

VA is an essential component of the life-sustaining therapy in end stage kidney disease patients relying on a sustained extracorporeal circulation for haemodialysis (HD) or haemodiafiltration (HDF) [1, 2]. Indeed, VA is often referred to as the lifeline or Achilles heel for a dialysis-dependent patient [3]. VA performance is a key factor to drive success or failure in all forms of extracorporeal renal replacement treatment [4]. Furthermore, VA dysfunction or complication is the major cause of morbidity requiring interventional procedures (angioplasty and revision) or hospitalisation [4–6]. Furthermore, VA morbidity represents a tremendous burden both for patient and health care system [7, 8]. VA management in chronic kidney disease patient is of tremendous importance in quality care of dialysis patients, since it represents a daily duty for care givers in the nephrology area to ensure success of renal replacement therapy, to improve patient outcome and to reduce burden of VA morbidity [1, 9].

2. Overview on VA management in dialysis patients

2.1 VA types

VA for HD belongs to three main categories: (1) arteriovenous fistula (AVF) made of native or autologous vessel (aAVF) or heterologous vessel (hAVF) [10]; (2) arteriovenous graft (AVG) made of synthetic polymer or bioprosthesis; and (3) venous–venous access consisting mainly in tunnelled central venous catheter (tCVC) inserted preferably in the superior vena cava system [11]. A schematic representation of various VA types is in **Figures 1** and **2**. aAVF is still the preferred VA strongly recommended by best practice guidelines due to its long-term patency superiority, higher performances and fewer complications in majority of patients [11–13].

Several autologous AVF types have been developed to fit with patient anatomic and physiologic characteristics. Briefly, according to their location on the upper arms, they are categorised either as distal (wrist) or proximal (elbow or upper arm); according to the type of anastomosis, they are categorised as side to side anastomosis or artery side to vein end anastomosis [14, 15] or vein transposition [16].

If the end-stage kidney disease (ESKD) patient is not a suitable candidate for an AVF, the AVG is the second VA option. Compared to the AVF, the AVG has better mechanical strength, earlier use, decreased primary failure rates, development of graft stenosis, a fivefold increase in infection risk, a poorer long-term patency, higher levels of complications and more interventions than AVF [17]. AVG should be preferred over a CVC because of fewer complications and better survival rates [18]. AVG access is made usually of synthetic material (e.g., PTFE) or biomaterial and realise a conduit between artery and vein [17]. Recently, a new biologic human acellular vessel, as a potential solution to AVG disadvantages, has been evaluated with promising evidence [19]. Human acellular vessels were implanted

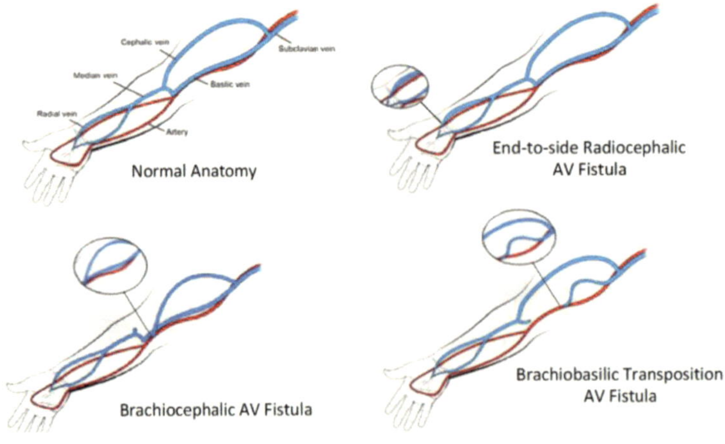

Figure 1.
Autologous AV fistula.

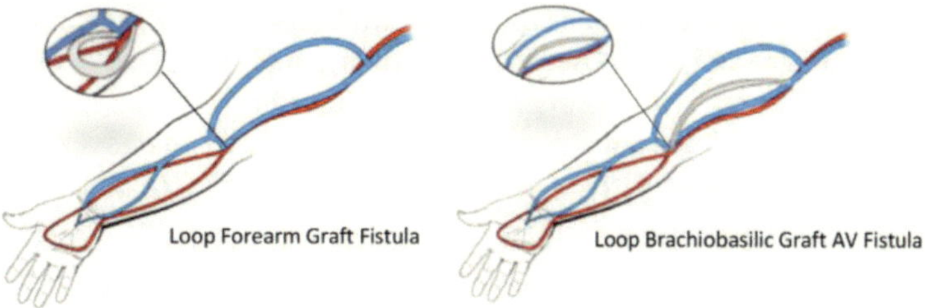

Figure 2.
Heterologous AV graft.

into 60 patients. The vessels had no dilatation and rarely had post-cannulation bleeding. At 12 months, 28% had primary patency, 38% had primary assisted patency and 89% had secondary patency [19]. AVG may be constructed either on the forearm as straight conduit (radial artery to cephalic vein), or as looped conduit (brachial artery to cephalic vein), or on the upper arm as straight conduit (brachial artery to axillary vein) or looped conduit (axillary artery to axillary vein). Less commonly AVG looped is created on the lower extremity (femoral artery to axillary vein) or as transthoracic conduit (axillary artery to contralateral axillary vein).

Although AVF is the preferred vascular access, double-lumen non-tunnelled catheter is the VA of choice when urgent or emergency HD is requested or when AVF/AVG becomes dysfunctional. Tunnelled dialysis catheters can be safely used as vascular access till the maturation of fistula and may be an alternative to arteriovenous fistula or graft for long-term VA if indicated. tCVC can be considered as permanent VA vein, in patients with recurrent access thrombosis, low blood pressure (cardiomyopathy), severe vascular disease ("steal" syndrome), trypanophobia (fear of needles), in case of premature exhaustion of veins needed for AVF creation and reduced life expectancy. Catheters are available in a variety of materials, configurations and tip designs, with the aim to maximise the blood flow, reducing recirculation preventing the catheter tip obstruction. There are well-established guidelines for selection of an insertion site for CVCs. The preferred site is the right internal jugular vein. In case, for different reasons, it is not possible to utilise the above vascular approach, and the second option is the left internal jugular vein. Other options are the subclavian veins keeping in mind the higher risk of subsequent stenosis or venous occlusion. The femoral vein for long-term CVC access should be avoided in patients waiting for kidney transplantation due the iliac vein risk stenosis.

2.2 VA prevalence

Interestingly, percentage of various VA types varies tremendously among HD population worldwide. Several factors contribute to heterogeneity of VA prevalent use and distribution that include dialysis vintage (incident vs. prevalent), age (young vs. old), gender (male vs. female), ethnicity, comorbidities (high vs. low risk), dialysis modality (HD vs. HDF) or dialysis setting (in centre vs. home or self-care).

Furthermore, it is of utmost importance noting that practice patterns have likely a strong impact on VA choice and prevalent use [20]. In other words, VA choice is not only driven by patient conditions or treatment modalities but also depends strongly on local or regional practice patterns including referral time to nephrologist, CKD patient management, care access, VA expertise and commitment, also patient choice. As an example, prevalence of AVFs in incident patients (<6 months) may vary from 20 to 80% from one country to another considering comparable patient profile, while the use of CVCs may vary from less than 5–80% in the same condition [20, 21]. Comparing VA repartition in prevalent patients, the same heterogeneous distribution holds true, with prevalence of 30% to over 90% of AVFs from one country to another with comparable patient profile [22, 23].

2.3 VA strategy planning

VA creation strategy planning is important to ensure best outcome to dialysis patients. It is now well established that careful clinical assessment and non-invasive vascular network mapping (US Doppler) facilitate VA construction and increase success rate [24–26]. Best practices emphasise and recommend such an approach to reduce failure rate and optimise VA creation, maturation and management [11, 12].

Early referral of advanced chronic kidney disease patient to nephrologist and to expert vascular surgeon may facilitate decision for VA choice and creation [27]. VA nurse coordinator has been shown to facilitate management of ESKD patients, to reduce CVCs use and to improve VA outcome in incident patients [28–30].

Few general rules for VA creation are recommended from best clinical practice guidelines: first, start with native AVF distal position at the non-dominant wrist and move proximally to the elbow in case of failure, second, favour artery side to vein-end anastomosis with reduced and fixed anastomosis diameter, third, consider using synthetic graft conduct in case of multiple failed attempts and fourth, tCVC might be a suitable option, in case of repeated VA attempt failures, in elderly patients, in patients with limited life time expectancy or as mid or long-term bridging solution to facilitate creation and maturation of AVF or AVG [12].

VA construction should be ideally performed within expert centres adequately staffed, imaging capacities and providing full clinical service to correct immediate or short-term VA dysfunction [31, 32].

2.4 VA performance and outcome

VA performance is crucial to ensure delivery of adequate renal replacement therapy. It relies on four main indicators: access flow, recirculation, pressure changes, and dialysis dose delivery. VA performance is more critical with short dialysis than in long or more frequent dialysis treatment schemes.

VA flow is the main parameter that drives dialysis session efficiency [4, 33]. Ideally, access flow with AVF or AVG should be higher than 500–600 ml/min to ensure extracorporeal blood flow of 350–400 ml/min. Choice of dual lumen tCVC should aim to achieve 350–400 ml/min blood flow on a regular basis [34].

In case of dialysis efficiency reduction due to VA dysfunction, that will be expressed by a Kt/V decline trend over time [35] (better if evaluated with online automated system and in continuous mode [36, 37]) and an increasing of serum potassium, phosphate, urea and creatinine levels. Dynamic pressure changes in vascular access either from venous or arterial side are reflecting VA dysfunction and suggesting a stenosis either on the distal vein or the proximal artery and impeding access flow reduction [38]. VA recirculation is usually very low and less than 1% with well-functioning AVF and AVG [39]. High recirculation (>10%) reflects VA dysfunction (e.g., stenosis of distal vein or proximal artery) and requires further investigation and intervention on VA if needed. It is important noting that tCVCs have by design and functional characteristics, higher recirculation than AVF or AVG. A well-functioning CVC has a recirculation closed to 10%, and higher recirculation is a strong signal of CVC dysfunction [34]. Recirculation is usually measured by dilution methods that sense either changes in US velocity

(Transonic) [33], electrical impedance, optical (CritLine), ionic dialysance change [40] or thermal changes (BTM) [41] with relative good concordance [42]. Fresenius Medical Care (FMC), Europe Middle East Africa (EMEA) and NephroCare (NC) clinics commonly apply the thermodilution measurements [43]. The thermodilution method makes it possible to determine the total blood recirculation with a non-invasive temperature bolus technique, and thus detect vascular problems that could reduce the efficacy of dialysis. This method can be used to assess both grafts/fistula and cardiopulmonary recirculation. In case the VA recirculation is confirmed the colour, Doppler US can provide an accurate anatomical and haemodynamic information, also measuring the access flow. This examination can be performed as part of a routine surveillance program, to detect early VA problems, or suspected dysfunction. However, limitations for its use are lack of staff and/or knowledge in the HD unit. Imaging techniques as the angiography and magnetic resonance flow measurements can allow a better definition of blood flow and stenosis visualising inside the vessel lumens.

In brief, reduced access flow, increased recirculation, low Kt/V and significant pressure changes are all indicating VA dysfunction that needs to be confirmed, explored and treated adequately [44].

A dedicated quality assurance program to VA monitoring and management is strongly recommended in dialysis facilities, as part of best clinical practices, to improve dialysis patient outcome [45] (see Section 4). VA outcome is usually best summarised by three hard clinical endpoints: functionality (e.g., maturation and access flow), technical survival (e.g. primary patency and secondary patency) and VA-related morbidity (e.g., dysfunction, infection and intervention) [46]. In brief, VA outcome depends on three groups of factors: first, patient medical profile (e.g., age, gender, comorbidity, diabetes and vascular calcification); second, VA type (e.g., autologous AVF and synthetic graft); third, practice patterns (e.g., creation skills, monitoring and maintenance) [47]. It is not our intent to review factors implicated in these outcomes but only to provide some brief trends and facts. Autologous AVFs have better survival than synthetic AVGs considering both primary and secondary-assisted patency [48–50]. Median technical survival with AVFs ranges between 3 and 10 years compared to AVGs which range between 1 and 4 years. Substantial loss of AVFs (10–30%) occurs shortly after creation due to thrombosis or poor maturation. Late stenosis or aneurysm may be observed with AVFs in long-term run depending on cannulation technique. Loss of AVGs occurs later due to stenosis in relation with myointimal hyperplasia in almost 90% of cases. Patency of AVGs requires tight monitoring and frequent restoring and maintaining procedural interventions (e.g., percutaneous angioplasty and stenting) [51]. Infection risk is about three times higher with AVGs. Intervention rate (e.g., angioplasty) to keep VA patency is 3–10 times higher with AVGs than AVFs in long run.

2.5 Complications in established VA

VA-related morbidity represents a tremendous burden for patient (pain, anxiety and depression) and healthcare system (hospitalisation, technical procedures and interventions and cost). VA-related problems represent a common cause of hospitalisation in dialysis patients accounting for 10–15% of cases [5].

VA complications vary according to VA type [52]. Arteriovenous accesses (AVF and AVG) are associated with less complications and risks as compared to tCVC [53]. AVF is still the "standard" for VA presenting significant less complications and longer survival patency than AVG [54].

Most common complications of recently created AVFs and AVGs are inadequate flow, failure to mature and thrombosis [55]. This aspect is further developed in the next section.

VA dysfunction in mature access requires further exploration and imaging (e.g., Doppler US, contrast media phlebography or arteriography and digital VA imaging) to identify the cause of poor flow or insufficient development. Based on the root cause analysis of the VA dysfunction, specific interventional procedures may be proposed. Usually they consist in percutaneous angioplasty with or without stenting. In the worst cases, surgical VA revision or new VA creation might be preferred.

Thrombosis occurs rarely as an unexpected event but usually follows and/or complicates an underlying stenosis of the distal or proximal vein or proximal artery [56]. This well-established fact reinforces the need for regular VA monitoring to correct pre-emptively this causal factor. Treatment of thrombosis requires urgent action by VA interventional expert consisting usually in a combination of thrombolytics and thrombectomy techniques [57–59]. After successful declotting, it is important to treat underlying stenosis by percutaneous balloon angioplasty to prevent thrombosis recurrence [60].

Aneurysms or more frequently false aneurysms may have developed on the vein segment of the VA either with AVFs or AVGs [61]. They result from repeated cannulation in the same area and high venous pressure. False aneurysms should be resected since they are exposed to further complications (e.g., infection and bleeding), and cause of high venous pressure (e.g., stenosis) should also be treated by balloon angioplasty.

Steal syndrome is a rare but painful and severe condition that needs to be treated adequately [62]. Steal syndrome results from retrograde blood flow after AV access creation, and a condition that diverts blood flow to proximal segment creates functional ischaemia in distal arm segment. It is more likely to be observed in severely arteriopathic and vascular calcified patients. Severity of steal syndrome is graded from minor (pale, blue and cold hand) to major (ischaemic pain, ulceration and necrosis of digits or hand). Treatment of steal syndrome consists usually in venous banding (high flow steal syndrome) or distal revascularisation and interval ligation (DRIL procedure) (normal flow steal syndrome). In worst cases, closing AVF or AVG would be considered as a safer option.

Infection of VA is not common in AVFs but more common in AVGs (2–3 times) and much more common (5–7 times) with tCVCs [63]. Infection results from specific risk of VA and chronic dialysis patient profile, but more likely from VA handling practices and hygienic rules of the dialysis facility [64].

Complications are associated with CVC placement (puncture of the associated artery, bleeding, major venous laceration, atrial perforation, pneumothorax and air embolism) and use (malfunction and limitation of dialysis performances, central vein stenosis or thrombosis and catheter infection) [65–67]. For patients who are treated with HD, the risks of major cardiovascular events, fatal and non-fatal infections and overall mortality are far greater with catheters than with AVF.

The NKF/DOQI guidelines define CVC dysfunction as the failure to attain a sufficient extracorporeal blood flow rate of ≥300 ml/min with a pre-pump arterial pressure lower than −250 mmHg [68]. Catheter dysfunction can lead to catheter thrombosis in the extreme. Early CVC dysfunction is defined as a catheter that never functioned adequately after placement and is mainly consequent to technical problems. Later, CVC dysfunction is related to partial or total catheter occlusions induced by intrinsic thrombus within the CVC, external fibrin sheath or extrinsic thrombus around the catheter in the vein leading to catheter adherence to the vessel wall or to the cardiac atrium. The majority of thrombi associated with CVC are asymptomatic. If the dialysis staff notices a decreasing Kt/V, an increasing level of serum potassium, phosphate, urea and creatinine and an increase of both negative arterial pressure and positive venous pressure during consecutive dialysis sessions, a CVC dysfunction could be suspected. If thrombosis involves the catheter tip, it may not be possible to withdraw blood and/or to infuse fluids and there may be leaking at the access site. In general, symptoms vary from local tenderness or pain at the site of entry to obstructive symptoms with swelling of the ipsilateral extremity, neck or face. Atrial thrombi may become symptomatic, with pulmonary or systemic (paradoxical) embolism or catheter dysfunction, or may be incidentally found as an atrial mass. In the experience of the authors of various studies, many patients who undergo an echocardiogram bring equivocal reports describing valve vegetation vs. tip catheters thrombi [69–71].

3. Vascular access creation and maintenance

3.1 Vascular access choice: selection bias

Whenever a native AVF can be created and is able to mature in no more than 12 weeks, it is considered the first and best choice as a VA [72]. Higher long-term longevity, less thrombotic or infectious morbidity, needs less procedure for maintenance. Overall a native AVF is big life and money saver.

The optimal VA is one that enables an adequate dialysis treatment, for as long as needed, keeping in mind that ultimately the natural history of a VA is failure. Its characteristics are a good blood inflow through the feeding artery, and an access flow (Qa) > 600 ml/min, without recirculation. It must be superficial (<0.6 cm skin deep), have a thick wall, a long straight segment to allow two needle punctures 2.5 cm away, a diameter > 0.6 cm, a good venous outflow, without causing distal ischemia in that limb.

That perception lead health authorities, some agencies and big provider chains to influence access choice through incentives and performance indicators, as if it was a black & white issue. In fact, AVF should not be always first and CVC are not always last. VA type comprises two of the nine quality metrics in the US CMS's five star rating of dialysis facilities a Quality Incentives Program (QIP) that rewards high AVF prevalence and penalises CVCs, without regard to patient case-mix.

There has never been a RCT comparing different VA choices regarding mortality or other hard outcomes. All large observational trials compared accesses achieved as opposed to the accesses that were intended (as in intention to treat). As 30–60% of all AVFs created either fail or need several procedures to mature and the CVC group in most studies were people in whom AVF failed, or CVC was chosen because of a predictable bad prognosis (old age, congestive heart failure, short life expectancy...), then we really cannot answer the question on which VA is the best or correlate it with hard outcomes [73]. If we exclude patients that begin HD urgently, mortality between AVF and CVC patients become identical [73].

VA is only one example of the paradox between patient-centred care and the tyranny of quality metrics based on population studies. Reconciling this paradox is what clinical judgement is all about and why physicians cannot be replaced by algorithms, care paths or protocol-driven medicine [74].

The native AVF comes with its own set of disadvantages. There is a higher risk of primary failure (non-maturation), up to 60% failing prior to ever being cannulated, angiographic procedures frequently required to assist maturation. Attempt to maximise fistula use by increasing creation rates has led to the unintended consequence of higher primary failure rate and longer dependency on catheters [75, 76].

Studies have shown that the primary failure rate is two times greater for fistulas (40%) than AVG (19%), with similar cumulative patency, in addition, the number of catheter days before AV access use was more than double in those having a fistula (81 days) compared with AVGs (38 days). However, grafts require more angioplasties (1.4 vs. 3.2 events) and thrombolysis (0.05 vs. 0.98 events) interventions per 1000 patient-days [76, 77]. The risk of primary fistula failure is much higher for lower arm fistula (28%) than with upper arm fistula (20%) [75].

According to the EDTA Registry, there is a trend for decreasing AVF in incident patients from 42% in 2005 to 32% in 2009, while there was an increment in CVCs from 58 to 68% (80% in the USA), with large international variation. In prevalent patients, AVFs went from 66 to 62% and CVCs from 28 to 32% [23, 78]. In a recent meta-analysis, CVCs (compared with AVF) have a higher risk of all-cause mortality (RR 1.53), fatal infection (RR 2.1), and cardiovascular events (RR 1.48) [18]. Grafts need twice as many angioplasties (1.4 vs. 3.2 events/1000 acc. days) than AVF, more thrombolysis (0.06 vs. 0.98 events/1000 acc. days). Although they need more procedures, their cumulative patency is the same when primary AVF failure is factored in [79].

Applying a proportional hazard model to examine mortality in incident HD pts aged 65–90 years old in association with the type of VA, but accounting for case-mix and health status, the RR of AVF is 1.0, graft 1.18, CVC transformed in AVF 1.2, CVC transformed in a Graft 1.38 and CVC permanently 1.54 (both adjustments reduce RR in CVCs of 44%) [80].

Using a decision analysis model (fed with data extracted from DOPPS 2, the REDUCE FTM study, the DAC study and CMS data) of the best option for patients initiating HD with a CVC, an AVF attempt strategy is associated with better survival and lower annual cost, but that advantage is progressively lost in patients above 60 years or diabetics [81]. The advantages of an AVF attempt strategy lessened considerably among older patients, particularly women with diabetes, reflecting the lower fistula success rates and lower life expectancy.

Although upper-arm fistulas have a greater chance of maturation, the loss of multiple lower-arm possibilities will sooner exhaust VA sites. Also, the upper-arm option exposes patients to higher frequency of steal syndrome, potential adverse long-term complications of high-flow AVF on cardiac function and an incidence of cephalic arch stenosis that is dramatically higher when compared with the forearm choice [82].

According to data from CMS, the first year cost in the common scenario of patients initiating haemodialysis with a CVC, the annual cost of access-related procedures and complications is higher in patients who initially receive an AVF vs. an AVG. In their first year, the average annual cost of an AVF is $10,642 vs. $6810 in an AVG. The CVC group had the highest median annual access-related cost of $28,709 largely attributed to high frequency hospitalisations due to bacteraemia, repeated use of thrombolytics, and frequent catheter replacement [83].

3.2 Timing of referral for vascular access surgery

It is consensual that once established, a native AVF is the preferred HD access, and all guidelines recommend placement of an AV access before dialysis initiation; however, that desideratum is achieved only in less than one third of all incident patients [84]. If we create it too early, the access may need extra procedures to keep its patency until dialysis initiation and many more CKD stages 4 and 5 patients will die of cardiovascular events than those who will progress to end-stage renal failure needing dialysis, and on the other hand, if we do it too late more than 60% of all patients will begin their treatment through CVC, without time for full maturation of their AV access [85].

Hod examined the optimal timing of incident fistula placement in a population of elderly patients above 66 years old, showing that the odds ratio for successful fistula use was maximised when surgery was performed 6–9 months before dialysis was needed, with worst results in obese females, in diabetics and patients with congestive heart failure [86]. Unfortunately, even when a patient is being monitored in clinic by a nephrologist, the rate of progression of CKD to ESRF is not constant, the need for dialysis can be precipitated by random, unexpected clinical events and the correlation between measurements of renal function and uraemic clinical symptoms are poor; therefore, it may be quite difficult to plan the best timing. The best strategy would be to develop techniques that speed fistula maturation below 2 months' time after surgical creation, what would make planning much easier and accurate [87]. Despite the tremendous heterogeneity in the decline of kidney function in stage 5 CKD patients, factoring in the presence of diabetes, the degree of proteinuria and the eGFR trajectory in the preceding year, significantly improved our prediction capability of dialysis commencement [88].

3.3 Access creation and early complications

Access malfunction is a source of tremendous emotional and physical suffering, dialysis treatments loss, low treatment adequacy, urgent need for a central catheter as a substitution access and referral for new angiography or surgical procedures.

The most common first VA complications include haemorrhage, usually at the sutures level, infection, revealed in the first 15 days, local pain/inflammation, failure to mature producing poor dialysis adequacy and early thrombosis. Non-maturation and thrombosis, both have as an underlying mechanism the development of early stenosis along the arterial inflow, in the VA itself or in the access outflow.

Stenosis is necessary for thrombosis, but it is not enough. Only 30% of stenosis above 50% of lumen compromise will cause thrombosis in the next 6 months, we just do not know which ones [89], and on the other hand, stenosis treatment based on morphology, percutaneous angioplasty, induces accelerated neointimal hyperplasia with recurrent stenosis [90]. In 20% of all cases, recurrent stenosis occurs in 1-week post-procedure and 40% in 1 month [51].

We define VA maturation by our capability to cannulate it with two needles and deliver a minimum blood flow to the extracorporeal circuit of 350 ml/min for the whole dialysis, 4 months after its creation, for a minimum of eight dialysis in 1 month [91].

Immediately after fistula creation, the blood flow increases from an average of approximately 20 ml/min in the radial artery to as much as 300 ml/min in a radio-cephalic fistula, 1 week later the mean blood flow rate increases further to an average of 540 ml/min and the mean shear stress from 5 to 10 dyne/cm^2 to 24.5 dyne/cm^2. Ultimately, the increase in flow in a well-developed fistula can reach 600–1200 ml/min [2].

The functional ability of the artery and vein to dilate and achieve a rapid increase in blood flow are the most important determinants of fistula maturation [92] and declared that success correlated much better with Qa one day after surgery than with preoperative vessel diameter [91]. Increased shear stress sensed by the endothelium, related directly with flow rate and inversely with vessel radius, initiates the vascular response and secretion of vasodilators and anti-inflammatory mediators, to reduce neointimal hyperplasia and lower shear stress back toward baseline levels.

At the pathogenic level, the stenosis seems to be caused by a combination of neointimal hyperplasia and an inadequate outward or positive remodelling [93]. The abundant presence of myofibroblasts within the neointima is consistent with a role for the adventitia as a source of cells for neointimal proliferation. New biologic interventions, delivered periadventitial during surgery may old promise in preventing fistula maturation failure [92, 94].

3.4 Prevention of early complications

The process of care to maximise AVF includes: (a) early referral to a nephrologist; (b) patient and hospital staff education to save peripheral veins, avoiding peripheral as well as central I.V. lines (in our experience, 75% of all patients in a renal ward have an I.V. line in the cephalic vein), as well as transvenous implantation of pace-makers to be substituted by epicardial leads; and (c) timely referral to the right surgeon (well trained and experienced in obtaining VAs), that will probably order, or preferably will do it himself a pre-operative vascular mapping. Remind him to avoid grafts, but, if no other choice, do not save in their length and that an AVF do not always have to be distal [95].

Preoperative physical examination provides essential information in patients needing AVF construction but is rarely sufficient nowadays because an increasing proportion of HD patients has a compromised vasculature, the result of age, diabetes, many years of dialysis therapy and prior HD catheters. Non-invasive assessment by duplex sonography is very helpful in locating veins that are not clinically visible and also provides information about their functional characteristics, including venous outflow. Duplex sonography is the method of choice for evaluation of arteries. A calcified artery with a small lumen and thickened wall will never provide adequate fistula function [96].

Vascular mapping (**Figure 3**) is a technique that leads to information on patient's inflow and outflow anatomy as they relate to arteriovenous access creation. It can be done by using US evaluation, or angiographic mapping, both have pros and cons, the choice depends on local expertise and availability.

The US scanner should allow examination with B-mode and Doppler mode, using linear array probes with a frequency of 7 MHz for B-mode and 5 MHz for Doppler. Patients more likely to benefit from pre-operative US evaluation are those with: (a) difficult clinical examination (obese, absent pulses and multiple previous access surgery); (b) possible arterial disease (older age, diabetics and cardiovascular disease); and (c) venous disease (previous cannulation) [97]. Doppler US has a distinct advantage of being a non-invasive modality that can evaluate both structural and functional aspects of vessels that play a key role in access maturation [98].

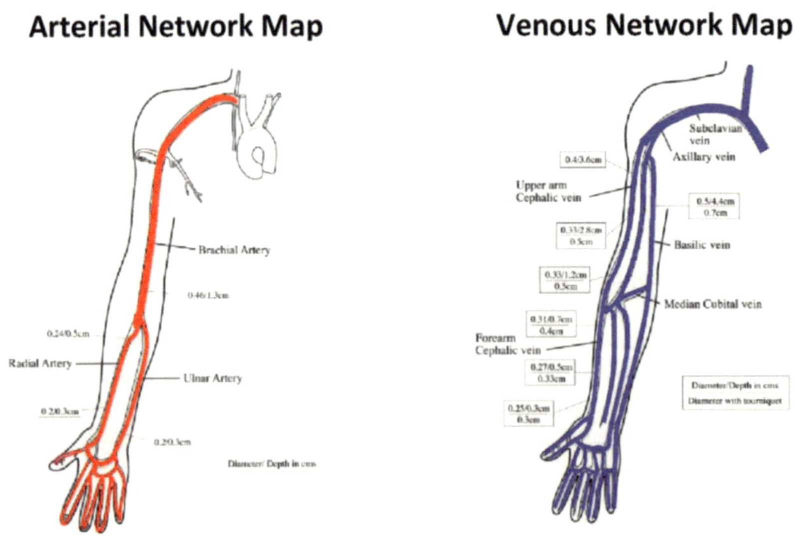

Figure 3.
Vascular network mapping: arterial map and venous map.

Preoperative mapping in some settings leads to marked increase in placement of AVF and a reduction in the use of catheters [24, 99]. Comparing pre-op US Doppler with physical examination, there was a dramatic increase in AVF creation 64 vs. 34% [24], reduction in graft placement from 62 to 30% and in tunnelled catheters insertion 24–7% [99]. Those were not universal findings, though.

The success rate of fistula formation does not correlate with vessel diameter but with flow, mainly in the day after [92], and in some series, a preoperative Doppler US achieved 80% successful constructed AVFs. Average parameters in this success cases: artery internal diameter 2.6 mm (vs. 1.6), Qa 54.5 ml/min (vs. 24.1), and resistive index 0.5 (vs. 0.7). Risk of primary failure is much higher for lower arm fistula, and long-term patency is not better, increase in vein ID after compression 59% (vs. 12.4) and Qa increased to 300 ml/min in 1 week (vs. 4–8 weeks) [100].

There is no systematic evidence that preoperative US mapping will induce an increase in the proportion of fistulas ultimately used for dialysis or a reduction in catheter use. It appears that the results from vessel mapping only influenced the decision as to the type or location of the AV access in surgeons with less than 15 years of experience [101]. In patients with pre-operative vascular mapping, on multiple variable logistic regression, factors associated with failure to mature were female gender, age > 65 years and forearm location (up to 78% if the three criteria were met), and the extracted mapping hemodynamic measurements could not differentiate patients with mature or immature forearm fistulas [102].

There is clearly more to maturation than vessel diameter, non-anatomic factors likely to contribute to maturation failure include the underlying vascular pathology and impaired endothelial function associated with CKD, vein trauma from surgical manipulation and the haemodynamic stresses resulting from the creation of an AV anastomosis [94]. Preoperative duplex US scanning and venography increased first fistula creation rate from 66 to 83%, but maturation rates actually declined from 73 to 57%, probably due to basing decision mostly on the vessels diameter [103].

4. Best VA outcome: role of a vascular access centre: quality assurance process

Dialysis VA outcome relies on three main components: support of a referent vascular access centre (VAC) providing expertise and service 24/7/365 per year; implementation of a quality assurance process optimising use of VA; commitment and skills of trained nursing staff ensuring best use and management of VA. This last part will be addressed more specifically in the nurse perspective section.

4.1 The vascular access centre in a dialysis network

A VAC is a dedicated department specifically designed and equipped to deal with VA dysfunction. Its goals are to provide easy access in less than 24 hours to an experienced VA surgeon or interventional nephrologist, to increase the prevalent number of patients dialysed through native arteriovenous fistulas (AV fistulas) and above all to reduce the number of patients requiring a catheter as a transient or permanent VA. Place and role of VAC are summarised in **Figure 4**.

The structure of a VAC is very similar to an ambulatory surgical unit, with continuous service from 9:00 am to 9:00 pm, 5 days a week, with a standard operating room and angiography suit functioning side by side, staffed by VA expert surgeons and interventional nephrologists. The perfect setup for a multidisciplinary approach to VA care is in a constant dialogue between surgeons and nephrologists.

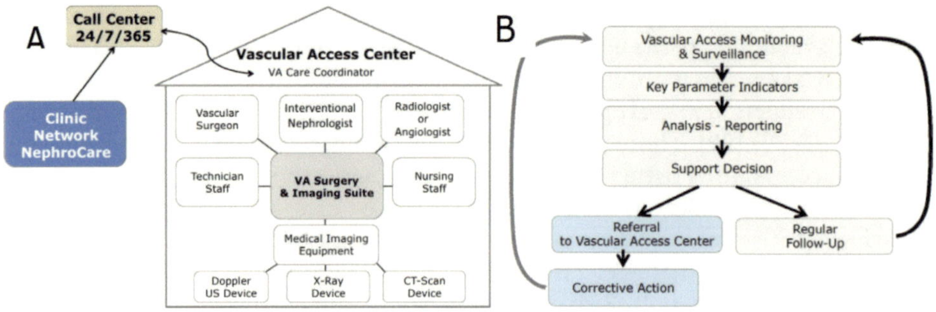

Figure 4.
(A) Place of VAC in clinic network organisation; (B) role of VAC in coordinating VA care.

The equipment should include a portable C-arm with capability for digital subtraction and road mapping, US equipment for central vein access localisation and puncture, pre-procedure patients´ triage and procedure planning, sterilisation facilities and a common recovery room for both disciplines. Supplies are tailored to operator preferences, within economic considerations [31, 32]. The VAC must be licenced by the health authorities, and their physicians credentialed to perform the needed techniques.

In our network, we manage around 5000 HD patients, treated in 37 dialysis units evenly covering the whole country, serviced by two freestanding ambulatory VACs and connected by a paperless dedicated software (VAonline©), a computerised database that handles dialysis unit referrals, reporting from the VAC back to the units and a permanent registry of our clinical activity used for research and administrative purposes. It connects and extracts data from the main network database (EuCliD).

Referrals to the VA are decided at the discretion of the attending nephrologist in the dialysis unit, and on arrival to the VAC patients are assessed to confirm referral correctness. Referral indications to the surgical pole of our VAC include: (a) construction and revision of AV fistulas or grafts; (b) exudative infection of the VA; (c) distal ischaemia of the access limb; (d) actively growing aneurysms; (e) haemorrhage or rupture of the VA; and (f) native AF thrombosis.

Referral indications to the angiography suite include: (a) graft thrombosis; (b) growing oedema of the access limb; (c) pain in the access limb during treatment; (d) unexplained reduction of dialysis adequacy (Kt/V) and/or VA flow (Qa drop < 600 ml/min in a graft, or < 400 ml/min in a native AV fistula confirmed in a second measurement); (e) SVC syndrome; and (f) native AV fistula non-maturation. Local bylaws require that all central venous catheters be implanted in hospitals.

Techniques performed in the operating room include: (a) construction or revision of native AV fistulas and grafts; (b) basilic vein transposition; (c) surgical treatment of VA infection; and (d) surgical treatment of ischemia or aneurysms of the VA limb. Techniques performed in the angiography suite include: (a) diagnostic angiography (mapping not achieved with ultrasound); (b) stenosis A=angioplasty; (c) pharmacomechanic thrombolysis; and (d) VA stenting.

In our series, with around 3000 interventions per year in both VACs, the most common referral cause is by far a drop in Qa in 61.2% of all causes, meaning that a VA surveillance program like ours, using daily physical examination by trained dialysis nurses and monthly measurement of Qa in the dialysis unit, although of controversial benefit, will have a major impact in the workload of the VAC and in the costs of the whole operation.

The most common site of stenosis, requiring intervention, was in the access itself in 31% of all cases, graft venous anastomosis in 29%, in the cephalic arch with

9.9% and the swing segment of the native AV fistula (the proximal segment immediately after the AV anastomosis) in 9.1%.

The most common procedures in the angiography suite were isolated balloon angioplasty in 67.5% of all cases, thrombolysis + angioplasty in 14.3% (depending on the graft prevalence in each region) and 10.1% did not need any endovascular intervention (false positive referrals). We decrease the implantation of stents, extremely expensive and not suitable for reintervention once suffering a stenosis recurrence, to less than 0.5% of all procedures, substituted in the same indications by drug eluting balloons. We were not successful accomplishing needed endovascular treatment in 7.1% of all cases.

Like the experience of others [104], in our centres, the procedures profile changed in the last years from a majority of interventions in grafts (angioplasties and thrombectomies) to one characterised primarily by angioplasties performed on AV fistulas. The number of interventional procedures did not decrease, and it was just the referral pattern and the percutaneous intervention required that changed in parallel with the increasing AV fistulas utilisation in prevalent patients.

A VAC needs a quality assurance program, to continuously monitor its performance. In our network, we use: (a) in first accesses an AVF construction in 80% of all cases; (b) in subsequent VAs 60% of AVF; (c) primary AVF failure at 3 months in less than 40% of all cases; (d) percentage of function VAs 7 days post-thrombolysis > 75% and at 3 months > 50%; and (e) absence of VA infection 15 days post-intervention. We also monitor the dialysis unit, requiring less than 1 referral to the VAC per patient year. We closely follow our success and complication rate according to international standards [105, 106].

In our experience, the major achievements of a VAC in our network are a substantial reduction in the waiting time for urgent procedures (28% of all referrals) to the same day response (elective referrals 4–6 days), the clear improvement of training and education of physicians and nurses in the dialysis units, now generating 0.3 surgeries/pt.Year, 0.37 angiographies/pt.Year, a precipitously drop of prevalent patients being dialysed through a tunnelled catheter from 24 to 14% and the total disappearance from our units of transient catheters. VA-related hospital admissions went from 1.3 to 0.6 episodes/pt.Year and they were 20% of all admissions and are now less than 10%. Our numbers compare favourably with the experience of others [107].

So, the question is, do we need a VAC for our dialysis patients? It depends on how good and how prompt is VA care offered in your region, if you are working in a capitated system, as in our case, is VA management included in the care bundle, are you mainly serving your own patients, raising the quality and coordination of care they previously received, or is there a market for you to sell a service outside your network. Do dialysis units in your area implemented a VA surveillance program, and in that case, do we intend to act pre-emptively to correct apparent malfunction?

To turn it into a success, it is important to monitor and influence the process of care delivered in our VAC, avoiding futile procedures such as AV fistulas that will never mature, diagnostic angiographies not needing therapeutic intervention (false positive referrals), useless angioplasties that will only accelerate more severe recurrences, or short-lived thrombolysis. It is imperative that we reach a consensus on how to define success and reward it (is it Δ Qa, Kt/V improvement, recurrence rate?). It is also of utmost importance to establish an accredited program for training young surgeons and nephrologists in VA care to guarantee future expertise in this field [108].

If we manage to be responsible for the full cycle of VA care, without sharing responsibilities with other providers, we may expect to keep costs control below the reimbursement rate, reduce the hospitalisation rate due to VA morbidity and limit the number of dialysis treatments lost. Reducing the number of patients with catheters we will avoid morbidity due inadequate dialysis, and the extra costs of supplies for in-treatment catheter handling as well the cost of thrombolytics to treat recurrent catheter obstruction and antibiotics to treat frequent catheter infections.

In the U.S. to break even a VAC in their current reimbursement environment, requires at least 800 patients, I suspect we would need a larger patient base in Europe; however, the feasibility of a VAC is quite variable and depends on unique payment structure in different geographic locations, specific needs of the patient population being covered and the availability of trained operators.

4.2 Quality assurance process

Patients with ESKD are fragile and vulnerable. For those who depend on HD, the ongoing success requires access to blood vessels capable of providing high volume extracorporeal blood flow to execute efficient HD treatments. Indeed, a properly functioning and reliable VA is one of the key successes of the HD adequacy. Unfortunately, the vascular access for HD continues to be referred to as the "Achilles Heel" of the HD procedure. Complications have a negative effect on the quality of life and continue to be a leading cause for morbidity and mortality of ESKD patients, with dysfunction being a major cause of morbidity and mortality in HD patients [109, 110].

VA options for HD include the placement of endogenous AVF, AVG and tCVC. The AVF is the preferred choice for chronic HD VA, rather than AVG and CVC, due the better outcomes (morbidity and mortality) and lower need for interventions and complications that could reduce both efficiency and efficacy of HD treatments which also increase the overall HD costs [111–114]. The selection of access should be individualised based on life expectancy and comorbidities and in consultation with a vascular surgeon with experience in the creation of HD VA. However, AVF is not always the ideal VA choice for certain ESKD patient categories such as the elderly: for those patients, the selection of VA should be individualised based on life expectancy and comorbidities. AVF, AVG and CVC are all used in older patients for permanent VA.

The HD VA long patency depends on several factors and minimises its complications, and failure has high priority in dialysis therapy and is a significant challenge for nephrologist, nurse and surgeon. The multidisciplinary team approach with agreement on a common set of targets [115], the surgeon experience [116] and adopting specific prevention measures such as, time referral for surgery with preliminary vascular mapping, specific VA surveillance strategies, AVF and AVG cannulation techniques with specific hygiene procedures are mandatory measures to prevent the VA both early and late failure or complications such as stenosis, thrombosis and infection.

The first challenge is the time referral to the vascular surgeon allowing to the AVF to mature adequately (1–6 months) and to be used for HD, remaining useable for many years with minimal intervention. Early referral of patients with CKD is strongly recommended. This approach helps to preserve access sites and provides adequate time for planning the creation and allowing maturation of the VA [68]. The most experienced surgeon of the HD vascular access team should be responsible, or supervise the AVF creation. Fassiadis [117] demonstrated that the primary success and primary and secondary patency rates of a series of consecutive radio-cephalic fistulae were affected by the experience of the surgeon. The risk of AVF primary failure related to ESKD patient increasing age, gender (female) and comorbidities (cardiac disease, pulmonary disease, peripheral arterial disease, diabetes and obesity) should be improved by careful patient evaluation and vascular mapping prior AVF creation. Patient evaluation (medical history and physical examination) and preoperative mapping of arm vessels allow a higher percentage AVF placements as well as an increased fistula success rate [24, 118]. Physical and US examination are intended to evaluate both the arterial and the venous system: vascular lesions, classified as inflow or outflow problems, should be identified allowing the surgeon the best AVF option protecting as much possible the arm vessel paucity for native AVF. The goals of the arterial evaluation are to find an artery capable of delivering the blood flow at rate to allow the HD treatment correctly. The axillary, brachial, radial and ulnar pulses should be examined as well as the blood pressure between the two arms to assure that the vessels are patent. By modified duplex Allen test is evaluated the hand arterial blood circulation if the radial or the ulnar arteries will be utilised in the AVF creation. The artery used must be of sufficient size (diameter > 2 mm) [119]. A forearm cephalic vein AVF (radial artery–cephalic vein) (brachial artery–cephalic vein) is preferred. The entire extent of the vein, its drainage, the diameter, depth and assessment of the ability to dilate should be assessed. The upper arm cephalic vein AVF (brachial artery–cephalic vein) is evaluated in case no suitable vein is found in the forearm. The non-dominant forearm is preferable for dialysis access placement, and the first choice used is the radio-cephalic AVF [111]. In case the first choice is not available, the other options from the most to least desirable are the following [113]: (a) dominant forearm radio-cephalic AVF; (b) non-dominant, or dominant upper arm brachiocephalic AVF; (c) non-dominant or dominant upper arm Brachiobasilic vein transposition AVF; (d) forearm loop graft rate; (e) upper arm straight graft; and (f) upper arm loop graft (axillary artery to axillary vein).

After AVF creation immediate thrombosis, failing to mature, or early fistula failure, may develop [120], and after the maturation late failure and other complications can occur [120]. VA monitoring and surveillance are crucial to ensure best outcome of VA and success to renal replacement program [121–123]. The AVF monitoring and the early identification of complications contribute to maintain the long-term patency of the AVF. Once the HD treatment is started, skilled nurses should evaluate the VA at each dialysis session. VA monitoring is performed on a regular basis synchronised with dialysis sessions to detect early dysfunction or complication. A routinely weekly physical examination of mature AVF is recommended by 2006 National Kidney Foundation Kidney Disease Outcomes Quality Initiative (NKF-KDOQI) guidelines and 2008 Society for Vascular Surgery [68, 119]. The nurse should inform the nephrologist in case of abnormal noise intensity [12], oedema, redness, swelling, bruising, haematoma, rash or break in skin, bleeding, other exudate, aneurysm or pseudo-aneurysm. The AVF blood flow is in the range of 800–2000 mL, and the thrill is associated with a blood flow >450 ml/min: in case the patient notices that the pulse or the thrill is reduced or it cannot be felt he/she should immediately inform the clinical staff. Patients should be instructed to keep the access extremity clean and to avoid wearing any cloths or wristwatches that restrict flow.

VA surveillance is intended to assess objectively and to follow over time VA performance and dialysis treatment delivery efficacy. It requires specific non-invasive tests and special instruments. Three main key parameter indicators are usually monitored: effective dialysis dose delivered, recirculation of VA [124, 125] and VA flow.

Time trend behaviour monitoring of VA performance based on selected indicators is crucial to detect early VA dysfunction (e.g., stenosis). Pre-emptive intervention has been shown very effective in correcting stenosis (percutaneous angioplasty) and preventing further risk of thrombosis and dysfunction. Precise knowledge of individual VA performances, threshold values (e.g., access flow

500–600 ml/min) and time trend analyses are required to optimise and personalise VA maintenance strategy [126, 127].

Time of first use or first cannulation varies according to VA type, maturation degree and local expertise: native AVF may be cannulated within 4–8 weeks after creation; AVG may be cannulated earlier 2–6 weeks; tunnelled CVC may be used immediately after insertion. Timing of VA cannulation (early <2 weeks or late >3–4 weeks) does not seem to impact VA outcome, and this is a particular feature of dialysis policy units [128].

The correct cannulation technique is mandatory for preventing AVF injury that might cause infiltration/haematoma or intimal damage with subsequent stenosis that might lead AVF thrombosis. Recommendations for the AVF cannulation procedures are few and mainly focused on needle size, angle of needle insertion and direction of needle bevel. Experienced dialysis staff only should be allowed to cannulate a newly created fistula. For first cannulations, local anaesthesia performed with topic anaesthetic cream or patch (Emla) is recommended [129].

In FMC EMEA NC clinics, the following cannulation procedures are applied [43]. The arterial needle should be placed in the direction of the blood flow and bevel down, but in case of anatomical restrictions, the needle is placed against blood flow and bevel up. The venous needle is always placed in the direction of the blood flow. The needle should be inserted at an angle of 20–35°, and when flashback is observed, the needle should be lowered and advanced into the centre of the vessel. Sites on the AVF which display evidence of aneurysm formation should be avoided. In mature AVF, 15- or 14-G needles are needed to support a blood flow rate of >350 ml/min needed for high efficiency dialysis or convective treatments. In 2006, NKF KDOQI guidelines recommended the use of arterial needles with a back-eye, to reduce the need for flipping or twisting the needle [68]. Parisotto showed in a cohort of 7058 patients from nine countries, that area cannulation technique (repeated cannulations concentrated over a small vessel area (2–3 cm)) was associated with a significantly higher risk of access failure than rope-ladder or buttonhole. Retrograde direction of the arterial needle with bevel down was also associated with an increased failure risk [130]. Moreover, patient application of pressure during cannulation appeared more favourable for VA longevity than not applying pressure or using a tourniquet [130].

The buttonhole needling is postulated to be associated with a reduction in haematoma and might increase long-term survival of AVF with less complication. The buttonhole technique is a cannulation method where the AVF is cannulated in the exact same spot, at the same angle and depth of penetration every time [131–134]. By using the exact same spot, a scar tissue tunnel track will be created. The procedure should be performed by the same cannulator until the track tunnel has been created. After track creation, this technique should always be performed by highly experienced staff. Using a sharp needle, it takes approximately 6–12 cannulations (depending on the individual patient) to create a track at a given site. The creation of a scar tissue tunnel track allows the use of a blunt needle [43].

The needle removal procedure is as important as the cannulation. Needle withdrawal must be done carefully in order to prevent tearing of the vessel, to minimise access trauma and to achieve optimal haemostasis. Each needle should be withdrawn slowly, keeping the same angle as that of insertion, until the entire needle has been removed. Digital pressure should be applied only after the needle is completely removed to prevent damage to the vessel wall and should be sufficient to stop bleeding but not so great as to stop the flow of blood through the VA [43, 135].

Cannulation and needle removal techniques are similar in patients with either AVF or AVG with the exception of the buttonhole technique that cannot be utilised to cannulate the AVG. It is suggested to avoid "flip" or rotate the bevel of the needle 180°. Flipping can lead to stretching of the needle insertion site, which can cause bleeding from the needle site and oozing, during dialysis treatment and can damage the graft [135].

Some medications, including statins, antiplatelet agents, anticoagulants, and dipyridamole have been reported to potentially affect VA outcome. Saran evaluated the association between VA failure and the use of specific drugs [136]. Calcium channel blockers improved the primary graft patency (relative risk [RR] for failure, 0.86; P = 0.034). Aspirin therapy was associated with better secondary graft patency (RR, 0.70; P < 0.001). Treatment with angiotensin-converting enzyme inhibitors was associated with significantly better secondary fistula patency (RR, 0.56; P = 0.010). Patients administered warfarin showed worse primary graft patency (RR, 1.33; P = 0.037). Statin treatment could be associated with reduced neointimal proliferation, vascular inflammation, and improved AVF dysfunction [137–139]. A Cochrane review reported that antiplatelet treatment can improve the 1-month patency rates of AVFs and AVGs [140]. Dipyridamole demonstrated to reduce ePTFE graft occlusion reducing the vascular smooth muscle proliferation and the neointimal hyperplasia [141].

Infection is the second most common cause of AVF-AVG loss after stenosis/thrombosis [9]. An effective hygiene and infection control policy is essential, and healthcare staff must be trained appropriately. Standard precautions prevent healthcare-associated transmission of infectious agents among patients and healthcare workers, and they must be applied to all patients. Appropriate sterile technique should be used [43]. The patient's skin must be disinfected with an appropriate solution (before needle insertion for approximately 30–60s) starting at the chosen cannulation site and moving outward in a circular rubbing motion. If the skin is touched by the patient or staff after the skin prep has been applied but the cannulation has not been completed, repeat the preparation.

The CVC exit-site infection can be defined as a culture-positive inflammation external to the cuff of the catheter and localised to the exit site and not extending beyond the cuff. It is characterised by local redness, crusting and a variable amount of exudate. In most of these cases, the patients respond well with local measures, like topical antibiotic application (without fever). The CVC tunnel infection is defined as a culture-positive inflammation within the catheter tunnel but beyond the catheter cuff, with negative blood culture. Usually it is characterised by erythema, tenderness and induration in tissues overlying the catheter and > 2 cm from the exit site. CVC-related bloodstream infection (CRBSI) is defined as the presence of bacteraemia originating from an intravenous catheter. The diagnosis of CRBSI is often suspected clinically in a patient using a CVC who presents fever or chills, unexplained hypotension, and no other local sign. Severe sepsis and metastatic infectious complications, such as infective endocarditis, septic arthritis, osteomyelitis, spinal epidural abscess and septic emboli, can prolong the course of CRBSI and should be considered in patients who do not respond appropriately to treatment. Specific connection and disconnection procedures to prevent the CVC infections are applied in FMC EMEA NC [69].

5. Patient perspective

5.1 Patient information and education

Patient information and education are powerful means for keeping VA functional and safe and to guarantee successful dialysis therapy. These needs extend to patient's family and relatives. Awareness and learning processes should start as soon as the patient is diagnosed with chronic kidney disease. VA creation is a significant milestone in the life cycle of CKD patient that marks almost the final step of kidney disease progression and announce the start of replacement therapy. VA planning and creation are usually associated with a severe psychological trauma in renal patient that needs to be adequately prepared. Therefore, regarding VA education, it is important to differentiate in the life cycle of CKD patient two stages: before and after VA construction.

Preservation of vessels is an essential message and task that should be given to any CKD patients and relatives [11]. It is of utmost importance that CKD patients are aware of how they can preserve their vessels in both arms. They need to realise very early that vessels are essential for VA creation as a line to life-sustaining therapy and superficial vein resources are not endless. Patient education should include information to avoid and/or to refrain using major vessels located in the forearm for blood sampling, intravenous (IV) injections and infusions or invasive arterial procedures and to avoid the use of upper arms veins for catheterisation (e.g., angiography) or radio-logical procedures (e.g., contrast media imaging). Such message should be repeated at each hospital or clinical admission. Instead the use of superficial veins of the hand and minor vessels of upper arm should be preferred for exploration or imaging.

Patient education means more than providing information, CKD patients will benefit from counselling to actively participate in the choice of their treatment modality, to act on their own care and in successfully self-managing certain tasks needed by their treatment [11]. Patient education is needed to increase patients' skills and confidence in managing their own disease. Education should be part of CKD management program during outpatient clinic consultation as a continuous training process. Long-term follow-up of renal patient gives caregivers and patient a better understanding of the choice regarding the type of renal replacement therapy and VA option. Obviously, patient education does not mean simply handing over information. Appropriate materials and personalised education (e.g., adapted to age, educational level, cultural and language barriers), that consist both in providing written documents, pictures, movies, social media and discussions, but also in regular checking of patient understanding and knowledge. This regular interaction between patient and care giver is one of the most efficient components of the educational and training process.

When the creation of VA is planned or performed, the patient must be informed about and what to be expected after the surgery. Also, he must be asked to report immediately to the VA reference centre if side effects or important changes occur. Important and practical advices after VA surgery include for example: to keep the arm warm and dry; to monitor the surgical wound for changes; to elevate the arm slightly to prevent swelling; to use the other hand to feel VA thrill; to avoid sleeping on the fistula arm, wearing tight sleeve, carrying heavy weights, violent sports or activity that may cause a trauma to the AVF; to avoid blood pressure measurements, blood sampling and IV injections on the VA; to ask dialysis nurse to check AV patency if patient is already on dialysis via a CVC.

Maturation of AV access is an important period for long-term VA outcome corresponding to the non-use of the VA. This time may last 4–8 weeks dependent on the VA type, medical patient profile and vascular network characteristics. After wound healing, patient needs to start appropriate exercise program for enhancing flow in the VA arm (e.g., open and close hand, squeeze soft ball and touch fingertips with thumb) that will foster VA maturation. Long-term monitoring of VA is needed for dialysis patient. In the patient's life, VA patency and local skin aspect should be checked at least daily. The easiest way is to put their hand or fingers on the fistula to feel a buzzing sensation (thrill) and to detect abnormal pain or temperature.

Patients with a dysfunctioning VA may require at some points imaging and/or interventional procedures. It is necessary to explain planned procedures or examinations to the patient. Patients should be informed about the contrast media use for the examination and be aware of allergy or other potential side effects. Expected results of investigation and potential required intervention should be carefully explained to the patient.

Hygienic rules should be applied any time on the VA arm to prevent skin colonisation and migration of bacteria from the skin to the blood circulation system at the time of needling (e.g., AVF or AVG) or VA connection (e.g., CVC). General recommendations consist in washing access arm with water and soap every day, before and after each dialysis session, avoid coughing or sneezing on the VA, keep the haemostatic and adhesive dressing for up to 3–4 hours after VA disconnection. Teach patients of the importance of preserving VA from special risky practices (e.g., sauna and steam bath, swimming, extreme sport and gardening with gloves).

5.2 Pain management of VA cannulation

Pain and discomfort caused by VA cannulation and needling are of major concern for dialysis patient. Pain assessment is a primary task and responsibility of nursing staff when caring dialysis patient [142]. Dialysis patients are exposed to pain with VA cannulation more than 300 times per year. Such repetitive exposure to pain and discomfort causes anxiety and depression, reduces quality of life, and interferes with daily life enjoyment.

Pain is an unpleasant emotional and sensory experience due to an actual or potential tissue injury that is tremendously enhanced by anxiety. This is a quite stressful condition that can lead to severe and uncontrollable fear of needles known as "needle phobia" or "trypanophobia" leading eventually to "dialysis phobia." In this sense, the pain control during VA cannulation by nursing staff should be considered as a top priority in dialysis units. Pain intensity during VA cannulation may benefit from regular monitoring relying either on subjective assessment (nurse feeling) or better and more objective assessment using visual analogue scale (VAS).

To prevent fear of needles and pain caused by the VA cannulation, dialysis nursing team should be adequately trained in pain management. Effective pain control improves patient satisfaction with dialysis nursing care, helps patient to accept haemodialysis and enhances their quality of life. Effective and personalised plans are needed to manage VA needling pain in dialysis patients. There are different pharmacological and non-pharmacological pain management strategies for VA needling. General approaches include topical heat or cold therapy, rhythmic breathing, distraction, transcutaneous electrical nerve stimulation, aromatherapy, acupressure, massage, active listening and music therapy. Topical treatment approaches aiming to reduce pain via local anaesthesia that include Emla (cream or patch) and lidocaine (cream or intradermic injection) or local analgesia such as Arnica topical cream or diclofenac sodium topical gel are now more frequently proposed. Other approaches may be advised such as hypnosis or gas anaesthesia with inhalation of nitrous oxide depending on the psychological component and on the local setting.

6. A value-based approach relying on best nursing practices learned from NephroCare

6.1 VA cannulation

VA cannulation method is still an "art" and procedure that reflects local unit practices and personal nursing skills [130]. Interestingly, despite the impact needling has on VA survival and patient outcome, there is no universal or standardised method proposed for proper cannulation [143].

There are three cannulation methods used by nursing staff: rope-ladder, area cannulation and buttonhole [144]. The rope-ladder (site-rotation) method appears to be the most used worldwide being considered as the safest one. It consists of alternating puncture sites at a defined distance from the previous one along the VA vessel as an attempt to prevent aneurysm formation, stenosis and repeated trauma by multiple punctures. The area (one-site-itis) puncture is the insertion of the needles in the same general area of 2–3 cm, session after session [145]. This method exposes to weakness VA wall with progressive dilation leading to false aneurysm. The buttonhole (constant-site) method is less used in centre but seems of great interest for patient self-cannulating their own VA. It consists in creating a track by cannulating repeatedly the same spot and angle with sharp needle over 6–9 weeks. Once the track is formed, then a blunt needle can be used for subsequent cannulation. Buttonhole cannulation appears to be less painful and create less anxiety than rope-ladder but exposes to a more risk of infection. Nursing vascular access procedures are detailed in a separate document accessible and downloadable from the website: https://www.edtnaerca.org/academy/publications.

6.2 Patients bearing chronic tunnelled central venous catheter (tCVC)

Despite strong recommendations from best clinical practice guidelines, the use of tCVC is very common and tends to increase over time in almost all countries either in incident (10–80%) and prevalent (2–48%) dialysis patients [20]. Such trend most likely reflects change in medical profile of dialysis patients (e.g., advanced age, comorbidities, short life expectancy and repeated failures of VA creation), change in medical practices (e.g., easy access to CVC and shortage of motivated vascular surgeon) and poor or fragmented management of CKD patients (e.g., late referral). Interestingly, prevalence of tCVC in prevalent patients varies from 20 to 40% in Europe.

6.3 Nurse perspective: skills, training and responsibilities

Nurses play a crucial role in the management of all VAs. VA assessment, cannulation and care are mandatory skills for dialysis nurses: failure to correctly perform this operation may result in serious complications for the patients [145].

6.3.1 Competencies and responsibilities

A highly-skilled dialysis nurse is required to ensure that each cannulation/connection procedure is carried out with minimal or no complications. At every dialysis session, and before each cannulation/connection, ensure that the patient's VA is functional and has no problems in obtaining the optimal blood flow ensuring an adequate dialysis [43]. The competencies and responsibilities to achieve this are as follows:

- The nurses should have competence in:
    - AVF/AVG and CVC assessment
    - AVF/AVG cannulation techniques and care
    - CVC connection and care
    - Management of complications
    - Patient education related to VA care
- The nurses should have responsibility for:
    - Ensuring patient comfort and safety
    - Reporting and documenting all complications relating to VA
    - Liaising with the dialysis medical team to early identify and manage complications

Before starting the cannulation procedure for AVF/AVG or the connection of the CVC, the Registered Nurse (RN) must assure the preparation of the environment, material and patient following strictly the hygienic rules.

6.3.2 Hand hygiene

The impact of health care-associated infections implies prolonged hospital stay, long-term disability, increased resistance of microorganisms to antimicrobials, massive additional financial burden, high costs for patients and their families and excess deaths [146]. In accordance with the WHO hand hygiene should routinely be performed.

6.3.3 Personal protective equipment (PPE) and work uniform

PPE (hand and face protection, aprons and gowns) serves to protect HCW from hazards and preventable injuries in the workplace. Some PPE items, such as gloves and masks, protect HCWs and patients.

Uniforms are not considered as PPE. Nonetheless they provide the HCW with professional attire that supports the HCW in carrying out her or his work in the dialysis unit, while at the same time preventing cross-contamination between the workplace and the home.

6.3.4 Patients general condition assessment

Prior to any HD treatment, assessment of patient's general condition to identify potential problems that may arise during the treatment should be performed: temperature (as a routine, only for CVC), diet, loss of appetite, vomiting, diarrhoea and any other intercurrences between treatments like cramps, bleeding or some other signs or symptoms of complications.

The nurse needs to weigh the patient and compare the value with the last post dialysis weight and to the prescribed dry weight. Blood pressure and pulse must be evaluated and all treatment parameters should be validated. When using a CVC, the catheter exit site must be examined thoroughly for the presence of any signs of infection. A physical assessment of the VA must be carried out before every treatment.

6.3.5 AVF/AVG assessment

Using the eyes, ears and fingertips, AVF/AVG are assessed for complications. Inspection (observe and look for):

- Signs and symptoms of inflammation/infection: redness, drainage, abscess, warmth, oedema and rash over the fistula.

- Infiltration/haematoma: needle infiltration of new AVF is a relatively frequent complication, and haematoma can develop easily in patients on chronic anticoagulation therapy.

- Pseudo-aneurysms are frequently seen on the fistula arm: pseudo-aneurysms develop because of trauma from cannulating the same site or due to a significant proximal stenosis in the outflow tract.

- Skin colour: changes in the skin colour could point to stenosis of infection, discoloured or cyanotic fingers could be an early sign of steal syndrome.

Palpation (touch and feel):

- Thrill: normally a very prominent thrill is present at the anastomosis and the fistula is soft and easily compressible, the thrill diminishes evenly along access length.

- Skin temperature: warmth could be a sign of infection; cold could be a sign of decreased blood supply (possible steal syndrome).

Auscultation (listen to the fistula):

- Listen for bruit: listen to entire access every treatment and note changes in sound characteristics.

AVF/AVG physical examination is crucial to evaluate the proper function and to detect possible signs of complications. If any sign of complication is present, the VA should not be used and the patients should be evaluated by the nephrologist [43].

6.3.6 CVC assessment

CVC, despite being considered the worst HD VA, is used in a considerable number of patients, up to 80%, either due to the need to start HD following emergency catheter placement or due to lack of native vessel to create an AVF or place an AVG. The goal of performing a HD treatment via a CVC should be the achievement of the best patient outcome as possible, while keeping all possible complications under control. For this purpose, it is fundamental that all team members are familiar with the principles of CVC care, which include assessment, usage, surveillance and maintenance.

6.3.6.1 Exit site

The exit site of the CVC must always be inspected at each HD treatment for any signs of irritation, infection or development of allergy to dress or disinfectant solution, including tenderness, skin peeling, rash, swelling, exudate and redness. European Renal Best Practice (ERBP) recommends to always ensure the area being cleansed around the exit site is slightly larger than the final dressing and include the section of the catheter that will be underneath the dressing [147].

6.3.6.2 Type of dressing

There is a wide variety of different types of products for dressing and securing CVCs, but the superiority of one over another has not yet been demonstrated. According to ERBP, for long-term catheters sterile gauze is preferable, for enabling maximal natural airing of the exit site.

6.3.6.3 Patency

Before starting the HD treatment, the patency of the catheter should be evaluated. The locking solution use in the previous treatment should be removed by withdrawing 3–5 ml, locking solution mixed with blood. Using a 10 ml syringe filled with 0.9% NaCl, a small amount of blood should be aspirate into the syringe and observed for clots containment. If yes, flush should not be done. If unable to flush the physician should be alerted to assess and, if necessary, provide intervention.

6.3.6.4 Patient's skin preparation for cannulation

Before needle insertion in an AVF/AVG, proper needle-site preparation should be done to reduce infection rates. Site selection should be done prior to the final skin preparation.

6.3.6.5 Cannulation

The most important procedure is the cannulation of an AVF/AVG, and over the course of a day, it is carried out on numerous occasions by the dialysis nurse. Choice of the correct cannulation site and technique are fundamental factors for an optimal dialysis session (more information at Section 6.1).

6.3.6.6 Needle taping

Tape the needle in place on completion of insertion, secure it using a minimum of three strips of tape: one to fix the wings, a second on top of it to secure the needle and a third one to secure the needle tubing.

6.3.6.7 Needle removal and haemostasis (HS)

The procedure of needle removal by the nurse is as important as the cannulation of the AVF. Needle withdrawal must be done carefully to prevent tearing of the vessel, to minimise access trauma and to achieve optimal HS. The needle should be removed using the same inclination as the insertion angle. Appropriate pressure should be applied after complete needle removal (thrill should be felt above and below the site of pressure). The pressure must be hold for 8–12 min without checking.

6.3.6.8 Haemostasis

HS of the first cannulation must always be performed by skilled nursing staff, since the vessel wall is fragile and there is an increased risk of haematoma formation. Manual compression applied by the nurse, health care assistant, or patient is the standard of care following withdrawal of HD needles. For the patients who cannot or are unwilling to hold pressure for sufficient time for HS the use of a HS clamp or band is required.

6.3.6.9 Patient education to care for VA

One of the most important responsibilities of the nurses is patient education. To achieve shared decision making, improve understanding and adherence, motivate, and encourage self-management, effective patient education is crucial [20] (more information at Section 5).

A good knowledge on VA management is necessary to enable the nurse to assess, plan, implement and evaluate the care given to patients before, during and after cannulation (AVF/AVG) or connection (CVC) and to deal with complications. The first use of a VA is an important opportunity for the expert nurse to demonstrate and transfer her/his knowledge and expertise to novice HD nurse. This will ensure the continuing education of healthcare staff engaged in patient care within the HD unit.

7. VA future outlook

As stated in the background section, VA is an essential component of a life-sustaining therapy in ESKD patients with a significant effect on both patient outcomes and associated costs [3, 8]. Therefore, taking a value-based approach and identifying opportunities for VA that would provide the right balance between optimal patient outcomes and total spending would be the ultimate goal [148].

The clinical/medical evidence basis clearly shows from a value-based perspective that it is obvious that native arteriovenous fistula is still the best VA option providing the highest survival expectation and the lowest complication risk [149]. However, patient profiles have become more complex including an increase of comorbidities that affect the success rates of AVF [150]. Therefore, several attempts have been made to substitute failing native AVF by new VA devices including vascular graft (synthetic and biomaterial), implantable devices (graft, venous catheter and port catheter) or hybrid system (graft port or venous port catheter) with limited success [151, 152].

What are the new VA perspectives to improve outcome and/or to expand VA possibilities in difficult cases. Several opportunities are currently under clinical investigation:

First, better management and use of existing VA from installation (VA network mapping) to maintenance permitted by use of non-invasive imaging (US-based) including monitoring technologies (online monitoring HD) [149, 153, 154] or connected technologies offering 24/7 continuous monitoring of VA patency [155]. The idea behind is to facilitate maturation of newly created AVF and/or to intervene earlier on failing VA to permit percutaneous interventional procedures for restoring patency [156].

Second, make better use and improve outcome of tCVC or implanted venous access port devices by implementing strict rules of handling and generalisation of catheter locking solutions [157].

Third, assess clinical value of minimally invasive procedures such as percutaneous creation of VA [158, 159].

Fourth, use medication either with systemic or local action to prevent thrombosis, to reduce neointimal proliferation leading to stenosis [160–162].

Fifth, evaluate performance and outcome of bioengineered VA conduit based on vascular matrix formation and autologous cell seeding as part of regenerative medicine [19, 163].

Next to the medical future outlook, the economic perspective should also be considered, reviewing the bottom part of the value-based healthcare equation where value "is defined as the health outcomes achieved per dollar spent" [148]. Two systematic reviews (one focused on VA creation and the other on VA maintenance) identified a total of ~15 economic evaluations and/or cost and resource use analyses. As from a medical perspective, AVF is concluded to be the most cost-effective VA type for HD patients [164]. Nevertheless, the number of studies identified, and the level of evidence currently available shows a clear gap in knowledge to come to a solid conclusion from a health economic point of view. Especially, the total patient life cycle with regards to costs is not clearly mapped including the identification of: downstream costs, costs of adverse events, associated costs of patency rates and long-term consequences in effectiveness of the HD treatment.

Finally, there is one additional component that would need to be tackled which is the health system set up in general around transition management for CKD patients including VA placement and maintenance. According to Porter, healthcare needs to be structured based on meaningful outcomes to patients to maximise the value that is delivered in the end [165]. As part of this structure, episodic treatment should be transferred to bundling therapies under the responsibility of one provider [165]. Translating this to renal care would entail to include VA placement and management in the dialysis reimbursement bundle, which is already the case in, for example, USA, Portugal and Spain.

The reason for this reorganisation is especially needed as currently approximately 32–73% of the CKD patient population experiences an unplanned start of dialysis [166–169]. This unplanned start leads to the use of the least optimal VA type (CVC) rather than AVF as this requires a 6-month maturity phase. This suboptimal start is caused by a lack of screening and diagnosis of CKD patients in time, as these patients are first seen by a general practitioner (GP) rather than a nephrologist [170]. Hence, awareness/educational measures toward GPs could also be one of the future outlooks from a health policy perspective to improve VA practice and consequently the lifecycle of HD patients.

In conclusion, the outlook for the future for VA practice is promising and has potential to improve significantly from multiple perspectives (medical, economic, health system, etc.). A collaboration and partnership between these disciplines would create an understanding and clear roadmap for next steps to put these into practice.

8. Conclusion

VA is an essential component of renal replacement therapy in ESKD patients. VA is currently referred to the life line of dialysis-dependent patient. Dialysis access relies on two main options: arteriovenous shunt (autologous AVF and AV graft); veno-venous access (tunnelled catheter and venous port device). AVFs are still the preferred VA option associated with best outcomes, higher performances and lower morbidity. Various innovative and quite interesting options, including minimally invasive percutaneous creation of AVFs and implantation of bioengineered vascular conduit deserve further clinical studies to enter in the VA armamentarium. VA performance is a key factor to drive success of extracorporeal renal replacement treatment. Furthermore, VA dysfunction and/or morbidity (stenosis, thrombosis and infection) are a source of frequent hospitalisation and corrective procedures. VA management in CKD patient is of tremendous importance in the overall quality care of dialysis patients. VA care and outcome are greatly improved in a large dialysis care provider network by means of a referent VAC and continuous quality improvement program [171].

Acknowledgements

We thank Jörg Rammo for conceptualising, designing the project and providing editorial assistance on the manuscript, Iain Morris for carefully reviewing the manuscript. All authors participated in critically revising the manuscript for important intellectual content and approved the final manuscript to be published.

Conflict of interest

All authors are employees of Fresenius Medical Care.

Author details

Bernard Canaud[1,2]*, Pedro Ponce[3], Maria Teresa Parisotto[4], Ellen Busink[5], Christian Apel[5], Jörg Rammo[6] and Stefano Stuard[4]

1 Department of Nephrology, University of Montpellier, School of Medicine, Montpellier

2 Medical Office, Fresenius Medical Care Deutschland GmbH, Germany

3 NephroCare, Fresenius Medical Care Portugal, Lisbon, Portugal

4 Care Value Management, NephroCare, Fresenius Medical Care Deutschland GmbH, Germany

5 Health Economics, Market Access and Policy Affairs EMEA, Fresenius Medical Care Deutschland GmbH, Germany

6 Business Development and Marketing, Fresenius Medical Care Deutschland GmbH, Germany

*Address all correspondence to: bernard.canaud@fmc-ag.com

References

[1] Beathard GA. Integrated vascular access management. Blood Purification. 2003;**21**(1):89-98

[2] Konner K, Nonnast-Daniel B, Ritz E. The arteriovenous fistula. Journal of the American Society of Nephrology. 2003;**14**(6):1669-1680

[3] Riella MC, Roy-Chaudhury P. Vascular access in haemodialysis: Strengthening the Achilles' heel. Nature Reviews. Nephrology. 2013;**9**(6):348-357

[4] Cortez AJ, Paulson WD, Schwab SJ. Vascular access as a determinant of adequacy of dialysis. Seminars in Nephrology. 2005;**25**(2):96-101

[5] Feldman HI, Kobrin S, Wasserstein A. Hemodialysis vascular access morbidity. Journal of the American Society of Nephrology. 1996;**7**(4):523-535

[6] Ng LJ, Chen F, Pisoni RL, Krishnan M, Mapes D, Keen M, et al. Hospitalization risks related to vascular access type among incident US hemodialysis patients. Nephrology, Dialysis, Transplantation. 2011;**26**(11):3659-3666

[7] de Kleijn R, Hagen C, Uyl-de Groot C, Pasker-de Jong P, Ter Wee P. Prediction of care burden of patients undergoing haemodialysis: Development of a measuring tool. Journal of Renal Care. 2015;**41**(2):119-125

[8] Jorna T, Methven S, Ravanan R, Weale AR, Mouton R. 30-day mortality after haemodialysis vascular access surgery: A retrospective observational study. The Journal of Vascular Access. 2016;**17**(3):215-219

[9] McCann M, Einarsdottir H, Van Waeleghem JP, Murphy F, Sedgewick J. Vascular access management 1: An overview. Journal of Renal Care. 2008;**34**(2):77-84

[10] Konner K. Recent developments in vascular access for hemodialysis. Saudi Journal of Kidney Diseases and Transplantation. 1997;**8**(2):113-118

[11] Schmidli J, Widmer MK, Basile C, de Donato G, Gallieni M, Gibbons CP, et al. Editor's choice—Vascular access: 2018 Clinical Practice Guidelines of the European Society for Vascular Surgery (ESVS). European Journal of Vascular and Endovascular Surgery. 2018;**55**(6):757-818

[12] Tordoir J, Canaud B, Haage P, Konner K, Basci A, Fouque D, et al. EBPG on vascular access. Nephrology, Dialysis, Transplantation. 2007;**22**(Suppl 2):ii88-i117

[13] Murad MH, Elamin MB, Sidawy AN, Malaga G, Rizvi AZ, Flynn DN, et al. Autogenous versus prosthetic vascular access for hemodialysis: A systematic review and meta-analysis. Journal of Vascular Surgery. 2008;**48** (Suppl 5):34s-47s

[14] Gracz KC, Ing TS, Soung LS, Armbruster KF, Seim SK, Merkel FK. Proximal forearm fistula for maintenance hemodialysis. Kidney International. 1977;**11**(1):71-75

[15] Wedgwood KR, Wiggins PA, Guillou PJ. A prospective study of end-to-side vs. side-to-side arteriovenous fistulas for haemodialysis. The British Journal of Surgery. 1984;**71**(8):640-642

[16] Rivers SP, Scher LA, Sheehan E, Lynn R, Veith FJ. Basilic vein transposition: An underused autologous alternative to prosthetic dialysis angioaccess. Journal of Vascular Surgery. 1993;**18**(3):391-396; discussion 6-7

[17] Akoh JA. Prosthetic arteriovenous grafts for hemodialysis. The Journal of Vascular Access. 2009;**10**(3):137-147

[18] Ravani P, Palmer SC, Oliver MJ, Quinn RR, MacRae JM, Tai DJ, et al. Associations between hemodialysis access type and clinical outcomes: A systematic review. Journal of the American Society of Nephrology. 2013;**24**(3):465-473

[19] Lawson JH, Glickman MH, Ilzecki M, Jakimowicz T, Jaroszynski A, Peden EK, et al. Bioengineered human acellular vessels for dialysis access in patients with end-stage renal disease: Two phase 2 single-arm trials. Lancet. 2016;**387**(10032):2026-2034

[20] Ethier J, Mendelssohn DC, Elder SJ, Hasegawa T, Akizawa T, Akiba T, et al. Vascular access use and outcomes: An international perspective from the Dialysis Outcomes and Practice Patterns Study. Nephrology, Dialysis, Transplantation. 2008;**23**(10):3219-3226

[21] Pisoni RL, Young EW, Dykstra DM, Greenwood RN, Hecking E, Gillespie B, et al. Vascular access use in Europe and the United States: Results from the DOPPS. Kidney International. 2002;**61**(1):305-316

[22] Pisoni RL, Zepel L, Port FK, Robinson BM. Trends in US vascular access use, patient preferences, and related practices: An update from the US DOPPS practice monitor with international comparisons. American Journal of Kidney Diseases. 2015;**65**(6):905-915

[23] Pisoni RL, Zepel L, Fluck R, Lok CE, Kawanishi H, Suleymanlar G, et al. International differences in the location and use of arteriovenous accesses created for hemodialysis: Results from the dialysis outcomes and practice patterns study (DOPPS). American Journal of Kidney Diseases. 2018;**71**(4):469-478

[24] Allon M, Lockhart ME, Lilly RZ, Gallichio MH, Young CJ, Barker J, et al. Effect of preoperative sonographic mapping on vascular access outcomes in hemodialysis patients. Kidney International. 2001;**60**(5):2013-2020

[25] AIUM. AIUM practice guideline for the performance of ultrasound vascular mapping for preoperative planning of dialysis access. Journal of Ultrasound in Medicine: Official Journal of the American Institute of Ultrasound in Medicine. 2012;**31**(1):173-181

[26] Gray K, Korn A, Zane J, Gonzalez G, Kaji A, Bowens N, et al. Ultrasound vein and artery mapping by general surgery residents during initial consult can decrease time to dialysis access creation. Annals of Vascular Surgery. 2018;**49**:285-288

[27] Astor BC, Eustace JA, Powe NR, Klag MJ, Sadler JH, Fink NE, et al. Timing of nephrologist referral and arteriovenous access use: The CHOICE Study. American Journal of Kidney Diseases. 2001;**38**(3):494-501

[28] Polkinghorne KR, Seneviratne M, Kerr PG. Effect of a vascular access nurse coordinator to reduce central venous catheter use in incident hemodialysis patients: A quality improvement report. American Journal of Kidney Diseases. 2009;**53**(1):99-106

[29] Dwyer A, Shelton P, Brier M, Aronoff G. A vascular access coordinator improves the prevalent fistula rate. Seminars in Dialysis. 2012;**25**(2):239-243

[30] Maddux DW, Usvyat LA, DeFalco D, Kotanko P, Kooman JP, van der Sande FM, et al. Effects of renal care coordinator case management on outcomes in incident dialysis patients. Clinical Nephrology. 2016;**85**(3):152-158

[31] Rasmussen RL. Establishing a dialysis access center. Nephrology News & Issues. 1998;**12**(6):61-63

[32] Rasmussen RL. Establishing an interventional nephrology suite. Seminars in Nephrology. 2002;**22**(3):237-241

[33] Krivitski NM. Theory and validation of access flow measurement by dilution technique during hemodialysis. Kidney International. 1995;**48**(1):244-250

[34] Canaud B, Leray-Moragues H, Kerkeni N, Bosc JY. K. M. Effective flow performances and dialysis doses delivered with permanent catheters: A 24-month comparative study of permanent catheters versus arterio-venous vascular accesses. Nephrology, Dialysis, Transplantation. 2002;**17**(7):1286-1292

[35] Mohan S, Madhrira M, Mujtaba M, Agarwala R, Pogue V, Cheng JT. Effective ionic dialysance/blood flow rate ratio: An indicator of access recirculation in arteriovenous fistulae. ASAIO Journal. 2010;**56**(5):427-433

[36] Badr B, Bories P, Marais R, Frat B, Seigneuric B, Longlune N, et al. Transonic, thermodilution, or ionic dialysance to manage vascular access: Which method is best? Hemodialysis International. 2014;**18**(1):127-135

[37] Daugirdas JT, Tattersall JE. Automated monitoring of hemodialysis adequacy by dialysis machines: Potential benefits to patients and cost savings. Kidney International. 2010;**78**(9):833-835

[38] Besarab A, Frinak S, Sherman RA, Goldman J, Dumler F, Devita MV, et al. Simplified measurement of intra-access pressure. Journal of the American Society of Nephrology. 1998;**9**(2):284-289

[39] Schneditz D, Krivitski N. Vascular access recirculation: Measurement and clinical implications. Contributions to Nephrology. 2004;**142**:254-268

[40] Mercadal L, Coevoet B, Albadawy M, Hacini S, Bene B, Deray G, et al. Analysis of the optical concentration curve to detect access recirculation. Kidney International. 2006;**69**(4):769-771

[41] Schneditz D, Wang E, Levin NW. Validation of haemodialysis recirculation and access blood flow measured by thermodilution. Nephrology, Dialysis, Transplantation. 1999;**14**(2):376-383

[42] Lindsay RM, Rothera C, Blake PG. A comparison of methods for the measurement of hemodialysis access recirculation: An update. ASAIO Journal. 1998;**44**(3):191-193

[43] Parisotto MT, Pancirova J. Vascular Access Cannulation and Care: A Nursing Best Practice Guide for Arteriovenous Fistula. 3rd ed. Hergiswil, CH: European Dialysis and Transplant Nurses Association/European Renal Care Association (EDTNA/ERCA). 2018. ISBN: 978-84-617-0567-2. Available from: www.edtnaerca.org/

[44] Besarab A, Asif A, Roy-Chaudhury P, Spergel LM, R P. The native arteriovenous fistula in 2007. Surveillance and monitoring. Journal of Nephrology. 2007;**20**(6):656-667

[45] Walters BA, Pennell P, Bosch JP. Quality assurance and continuous quality improvement programs for vascular access care. Contributions to Nephrology. 2004;**142**:323-349

[46] Viecelli AK, O'Lone E, Sautenet B, Craig JC, Tong A, Chemla E, et al. Vascular access outcomes reported in maintenance hemodialysis trials: A systematic review. American Journal of Kidney Diseases. 2018;**71**(3):382-391

[47] Smith GE, Gohil R, Chetter IC. Factors affecting the patency of arteriovenous fistulas for dialysis

access. Journal of Vascular Surgery. 2012;**55**(3):849-855

[48] Gibson KD, Gillen DL, Caps MT, Kohler TR, Sherrard DJ, Stehman-Breen CO. Vascular access survival and incidence of revisions: A comparison of prosthetic grafts, simple autogenous fistulas, and venous transposition fistulas from the United States Renal Data System Dialysis Morbidity and Mortality Study. Journal of Vascular Surgery. 2001;**34**(4):694-700

[49] Harms JC, Rangarajan S, Young CJ, Barker-Finkel J, Allon M. Outcomes of arteriovenous fistulas and grafts with or without intervention before successful use. Journal of Vascular Surgery. 2016;**64**(1):155-162

[50] Almasri J, Alsawas M, Mainou M, Mustafa RA, Wang Z, Woo K, et al. Outcomes of vascular access for hemodialysis: A systematic review and meta-analysis. Journal of Vascular Surgery. 2016;**64**(1):236-243

[51] Moist LM, Churchill DN, House AA, Millward SF, Elliott JE, Kribs SW, et al. Regular monitoring of access flow compared with monitoring of venous pressure fails to improve graft survival. Journal of the American Society of Nephrology. 2003;**14**(10):2645-2653

[52] Al-Jaishi AA, Liu AR, Lok CE, Zhang JC, Moist LM. Complications of the arteriovenous fistula: A systematic review. Journal of the American Society of Nephrology. 2017;**28**(6):1839-1850

[53] Padberg FT Jr, Calligaro KD, Sidawy AN. Complications of arteriovenous hemodialysis access: Recognition and management. Journal of Vascular Surgery. 2008;**48**(Suppl 5): 55S-80S

[54] Leapman SB, Boyle M, Pescovitz MD, Milgrom ML, Jindal RM, Filo RS. The arteriovenous fistula for hemodialysis access: Gold standard or archaic relic? The American Surgeon. 1996;**62**(8):652-656; discussion 6-7

[55] Stolic R. Most important chronic complications of arteriovenous fistulas for hemodialysis. Medical Principles and Practice. 2013;**22**(3):220-228

[56] MacRae JM, Dipchand C, Oliver M, Moist L, Lok C, Clark E, et al. Arteriovenous access failure, stenosis, and thrombosis. Canadian Journal of Kidney Health and Disease. 2016:3-11

[57] Turmel-Rodrigues LA. Hemodialysis access declotting: A native fistula is not a prosthetic graft. Journal of Vascular and Interventional Radiology. 2000;**11**(1):135-137

[58] Beathard GA. Does stenting prolong the patency of arteriovenous grafts after thrombectomy and angioplasty? Nature Clinical Practice. Nephrology. 2006;**2**(10):554-555

[59] Haage P, Gunther RW. Radiological intervention to maintain vascular access. European Journal of Vascular and Endovascular Surgery. 2006;**32**(1):84-89

[60] Bountouris I, Kritikou G, Degermetzoglou N, Avgerinos KI. A review of percutaneous transluminal angioplasty in hemodialysis fistula. International Journal of Vascular Medicine. 2018;**2018**:1420136

[61] Inston N, Mistry H, Gilbert J, Kingsmore D, Raza Z, Tozzi M, et al. Aneurysms in vascular access: State of the art and future developments. The Journal of Vascular Access. 2017;**18**(6):464-472

[62] Malik J, Tuka V, Kasalova Z, Chytilova E, Slavikova M, Clagett P, et al. Understanding the dialysis access steal syndrome. A review of the etiologies, diagnosis, prevention and treatment strategies. The Journal of Vascular Access. 2018;**9**(3):155-166

[63] Hoen B, Paul-Dauphin A, Hestin D, Kessler M. EPIBACDIAL: A multicenter prospective study of risk factors for bacteremia in chronic hemodialysis patients. Journal of the American Society of Nephrology. 1998;**9**(5):869-876

[64] Nassar GM, Ayus JC. Infectious complications of the hemodialysis access. Kidney International. 2001;**60**(1):1-13

[65] Saad TF. Bacteremia associated with tunneled, cuffed hemodialysis catheters. American Journal of Kidney Diseases. 1999;**34**(6):1114-1124

[66] Beathard GA. Dysfunction of new catheters by old fibrin sheaths. Seminars in Dialysis. 2004;**17**(3):243-244

[67] MacRae JM, Ahmed A, Johnson N, Levin A, Kiaii M. Central vein stenosis: A common problem in patients on hemodialysis. ASAIO Journal. 2005;**51**(1):77-81

[68] Vascular Access Work G. Clinical practice guidelines for vascular access. American Journal of Kidney Diseases. 2006;**48**(Suppl 1):S176-S247

[69] Parisotto MT, Pinto B, Miriunis C, Pelliccia F, Morris I, Romach I, et al. Vascular Access Management and Care: A Nursing Best Practice Guide for Central Venous Catheter. 1st ed. Hergiswil, CH: European Dialysis and Transplant Nurses Association/European Renal Care Association (EDTNA/ERCA); 2018. ISBN: 978-84-09-04228-9

[70] Rooden CJ, Tesselaar ME, Osanto S, Rosendaal FR, Huisman MV. Deep vein thrombosis associated with central venous catheters—A review. Journal of Thrombosis and Haemostasis. 2005;**3**(11):2409-2419

[71] Liangos O, Gul A, Madias NE, Jaber BL. Long-term management of the tunneled venous catheter. Seminars in Dialysis. 2006;**19**(2):158-164

[72] Biuckians A, Scott EC, Meier GH, Panneton JM, Glickman MH. The natural history of autologous fistulas as first-time dialysis access in the KDOQI era. Journal of Vascular Surgery. 2008;**47**(2):415-421; discussion 20-1

[73] Quinn RR, Ravani P. Fistula-first and catheter-last: Fading certainties and growing doubts. Nephrology, Dialysis, Transplantation. 2014;**29**(4):727-730

[74] Wish JB. Catheter last, fistula not-so-first. Journal of the American Society of Nephrology. 2015;**26**(1):5-7

[75] Al-Jaishi AA, Oliver MJ, Thomas SM, Lok CE, Zhang JC, Garg AX, et al. Patency rates of the arteriovenous fistula for hemodialysis: A systematic review and meta-analysis. American Journal of Kidney Diseases. 2014;**63**(3):464-478

[76] Lok CE, Sontrop JM, Tomlinson G, Rajan D, Cattral M, Oreopoulos G, et al. Cumulative patency of contemporary fistulas versus grafts (2000-2010). Clinical Journal of the American Society of Nephrology. 2013;**8**(5):810-818

[77] Al-Jaishi AA, Moist LM. Fistula eligibility: A work in progress. Seminars in Dialysis. 2014;**27**(2):173-178

[78] Noordzij M, Jager KJ, van der Veer SN, Kramar R, Collart F, Heaf JG, et al. Use of vascular access for haemodialysis in Europe: A report from the ERA-EDTA Registry. Nephrology, Dialysis, Transplantation. 2014;**29**(10):1956-1964

[79] Allon M, Lok CE. Dialysis fistula or graft: The role for randomized clinical trials. Clinical Journal of the American Society of Nephrology. 2010;**5**(12):2348-2354

[80] Grubbs V, Wasse H, Vittinghoff E, Grimes BA, Johansen KL. Health

status as a potential mediator of the association between hemodialysis vascular access and mortality. Nephrology, Dialysis, Transplantation. 2014;**29**(4):892-898

[81] Drew DA, Lok CE, Cohen JT, Wagner M, Tangri N, Weiner DE. Vascular access choice in incident hemodialysis patients: A decision analysis. Journal of the American Society of Nephrology. 2015;**26**(1):183-191

[82] Amerling R, Ronco C, Kuhlman M, Winchester JF. Arteriovenous fistula toxicity. Blood Purification. 2011;**31**(1-3):113-120

[83] Al-Balas A, Lee T, Young CJ, Kepes JA, Barker-Finkel J, Allon M. The clinical and economic effect of vascular access selection in patients initiating hemodialysis with a catheter. Journal of the American Society of Nephrology. 2017;**28**(12):3679-3687

[84] Stehman-Breen CO, Sherrard DJ, Gillen D, Caps M. Determinants of type and timing of initial permanent hemodialysis vascular access. Kidney International. 2000;**57**(2):639-645

[85] Collins AJ, Foley RN, Chavers B, Gilbertson D, Herzog C, Ishani A, et al. US renal data system 2013 annual data report. American Journal of Kidney Diseases. 2014;**63**(Suppl 1):A7

[86] Hod T, Patibandla BK, Vin Y, Brown RS, Goldfarb-Rumyantzev AS. Arteriovenous fistula placement in the elderly: When is the optimal time? Journal of the American Society of Nephrology. 2015;**26**(2):448-456

[87] Dixon BS. Timing of arteriovenous fistula placement: Keeping it in perspective. Journal of the American Society of Nephrology. 2015;**26**(2):241-243

[88] Al-Balas A, Lee T, Young CJ, Barker-Finkel J, Allon M. Predictors of initiation for predialysis arteriovenous fistula. Clinical Journal of the American Society of Nephrology. 2016;**11**(10):1802-1808

[89] Lumsden AB, MacDonald MJ, Kikeri D, Cotsonis GA, Harker LA, Martin LG. Prophylactic balloon angioplasty fails to prolong the patency of expanded polytetrafluoroethylene arteriovenous grafts: Results of a prospective randomized study. Journal of Vascular Surgery. 1997;**26**(3): 382-390; discussion 90-2

[90] Chang CJ, Ko PJ, Hsu LA, Ko YS, Ko YL, Chen CF, et al. Highly increased cell proliferation activity in the restenotic hemodialysis vascular access after percutaneous transluminal angioplasty: Implication in prevention of restenosis. American Journal of Kidney Diseases. 2004;**43**(1):74-84

[91] Achneck HE, Sileshi B, Li M, Partington EJ, Peterson DA, Lawson JH. Surgical aspects and biological considerations of arteriovenous fistula placement. Seminars in Dialysis. 2010;**23**(1):25-33

[92] Dixon BS. Why don't fistulas mature? Kidney International. 2006;**70**(8):1413-1422

[93] Roy-Chaudhury P. Pragmatic, precision medicine approaches for dialysis vascular access dysfunction: Challenges and opportunities. Clinical Journal of the American Society of Nephrology. 2016;**11**(9):1525-1526

[94] Dember LM, Dixon BS. Early fistula failure: Back to basics. American Journal of Kidney Diseases. 2007;**50**(5):696-699

[95] Choi KL, Salman L, Krishnamurthy G, Mercado C, Merrill D, Thomas I, et al. Impact of surgeon selection on access placement and survival following preoperative mapping in the

"Fistula First" era. Seminars in Dialysis. 2008;**21**(4):341-345

[96] Malovrh M. The role of sonography in the planning of arteriovenous fistulas for hemodialysis. Seminars in Dialysis. 2003;**16**(4):299-303

[97] Ferring M, Henderson J, Wilmink A, Smith S. Vascular ultrasound for the pre-operative evaluation prior to arteriovenous fistula formation for haemodialysis: Review of the evidence. Nephrology, Dialysis, Transplantation. 2008;**23**(6):1809-1815

[98] Wilson NA, Shenoy S. Ultrasound in preoperative evaluation for dialysis-access placement. Seminars in Dialysis. 2014;**27**(6):593-595

[99] Silva MB Jr, Hobson RW 2nd, Pappas PJ, Jamil Z, Araki CT, Goldberg MC, et al. A strategy for increasing use of autogenous hemodialysis access procedures: Impact of preoperative noninvasive evaluation. Journal of Vascular Surgery. 1998;**27**(2):302-307; discussion 7-8

[100] Malovrh M. Native arteriovenous fistula: Preoperative evaluation. American Journal of Kidney Diseases. 2002;**39**(6):1218-1225

[101] Nica A, Lok CE, Harris J, Lee TC, Mokrzycki MH, Maya ID, et al. Understanding surgical preference and practice in hemodialysis vascular access creation. Seminars in Dialysis. 2013;**26**(4):520-526

[102] Peterson WJ, Barker J, Allon M. Disparities in fistula maturation persist despite preoperative vascular mapping. Clinical Journal of the American Society of Nephrology. 2008;**3**(2):437-441

[103] Patel ST, Hughes J, Mills JL Sr. Failure of arteriovenous fistula maturation: An unintended consequence of exceeding dialysis outcome quality Initiative guidelines for hemodialysis access. Journal of Vascular Surgery. 2003;**38**(3):439-445; discussion 45

[104] Beathard GA, Urbanes A, Litchfield T. Changes in the profile of endovascular procedures performed in freestanding dialysis access centers over 15 years. Clinical Journal of the American Society of Nephrology. 2017;**12**(5):779-786

[105] Vesely TM, Beathard G, Ash S, Hoggard J, Schon D. Classification of complications associated with hemodialysis vascular access procedures. A position statement from the American Society of Diagnostic and Interventional Nephrology. The Journal of Vascular Access. 2008;**9**(1):12-19

[106] Beathard GA. Management of complications of endovascular dialysis access procedures. Seminars in Dialysis. 2003;**16**(4):309-313

[107] Mishler R, Sands JJ, Ofsthun NJ, Teng M, Schon D, Lazarus JM. Dedicated outpatient vascular access center decreases hospitalization and missed outpatient dialysis treatments. Kidney International. 2006;**69**(2):393-398

[108] Saad TF. Training, certification, and reimbursement for nephrology procedures. Seminars in Nephrology. 2002;**22**(3):276-285

[109] Dhingra RK, Young EW, Hulbert-Shearon TE, Leavey SF, Port FK. Type of vascular access and mortality in U.S. hemodialysis patients. Kidney International. 2001;**60**(4):1443-1451

[110] Pisoni RL, Arrington CJ, Albert JM, Ethier J, Kimata N, Krishnan M, et al. Facility hemodialysis vascular access use and mortality in countries participating in DOPPS: An instrumental variable analysis. American Journal of Kidney Diseases. 2009;**53**(3):475-491

[111] Hemodialysis Adequacy Work G. Clinical practice guidelines for hemodialysis adequacy, update 2006. American Journal of Kidney Diseases. 2006;**48**(Suppl 1):S2-S90

[112] Huber TS, Carter JW, Carter RL, Seeger JM. Patency of autogenous and polytetrafluoroethylene upper extremity arteriovenous hemodialysis accesses: A systematic review. Journal of Vascular Surgery. 2003;**38**(5):1005-1011

[113] Allon M, Robbin ML. Increasing arteriovenous fistulas in hemodialysis patients: Problems and solutions. Kidney International. 2002;**62**(4):1109-1124

[114] Farber A, Imrey PB, Huber TS, Kaufman JM, Kraiss LW, Larive B, et al. Multiple preoperative and intraoperative factors predict early fistula thrombosis in the Hemodialysis Fistula Maturation Study. Journal of Vascular Surgery. 2016;**63**(1):163-170 e6

[115] Allon M, Bailey R, Ballard R, Deierhoi MH, Hamrick K, Oser R, et al. A multidisciplinary approach to hemodialysis access: Prospective evaluation. Kidney International. 1998;**53**(2):473-479

[116] Dixon BS, Novak L, Fangman J. Hemodialysis vascular access survival: Upper-arm native arteriovenous fistula. American Journal of Kidney Diseases. 2002;**39**(1):92-101

[117] Fassiadis N, Morsy M, Siva M, Marsh JE, Makanjuola AD, Chemla ES. Does the surgeon's experience impact on radiocephalic fistula patency rates? Seminars in Dialysis. 2007;**20**(5):455-457

[118] Wong CS, McNicholas N, Healy D, Clarke-Moloney M, Coffey JC, Grace PA, et al. A systematic review of preoperative duplex ultrasonography and arteriovenous fistula formation. Journal of Vascular Surgery. 2013;**57**(4):1129-1133

[119] Sidawy AN, Spergel LM, Besarab A, Allon M, Jennings WC, Padberg FT Jr, et al. The society for vascular surgery: Clinical practice guidelines for the surgical placement and maintenance of arteriovenous hemodialysis access. Journal of Vascular Surgery. 2008;**48**(Suppl 5):2S-25S

[120] Mercado C, Salman L, Krishnamurthy G, Choi K, Artikov S, Thomas I, et al. Early and late fistula failure. Clinical Nephrology. 2008;**69**(2):77-83

[121] Vanholder R. Vascular access: Care and monitoring of function. Nephrology, Dialysis, Transplantation. 2001;**16**(8):1542-1545

[122] Pengloan J. Vascular access: Care and monitoring. Nephrology, Dialysis, Transplantation. 2002;**17**(6):1141-1142; author reply 2-5

[123] Haddad NJ, Winoto J, Shidham G, Agarwal AK. Hemodialysis access monitoring and surveillance, how and why? Frontiers in Bioscience (Elite Edition). 2012;**4**:2396-2401

[124] Paulson WD, Gadallah MF, Bieber BJ, Altman SD, Birk CG, Work J. Accuracy and reproducibility of urea recirculation in detecting haemodialysis access stenosis. Nephrology, Dialysis, Transplantation. 1998;**13**(1):118-124

[125] Schneditz D. Theoretical and practical issues in recirculation: Assessment of vascular access. EDTNA/ERCA Journal. 1998;**24**(2):3-6

[126] Paulson WD, Ram SJ, Birk CG, Work J. Does blood flow accurately predict thrombosis or failure of hemodialysis synthetic grafts? A meta-analysis. American Journal of Kidney Diseases. 1999;**34**(3):478-485

[127] Paulson WD, Ram SJ, Birk CG, Zapczynski M, Martin SR, Work J.

Accuracy of decrease in blood flow in predicting hemodialysis graft thrombosis. American Journal of Kidney Diseases. 2000;**35**(6):1089-1095

[128] Saran R, Dykstra DM, Pisoni RL, Akiba T, Akizawa T, Canaud B, et al. Timing of first cannulation and vascular access failure in haemodialysis: An analysis of practice patterns at dialysis facilities in the DOPPS. Nephrology, Dialysis, Transplantation. 2004;**19**(9):2334-2340

[129] George P, Masih D, Philip N, Shelly D, Rajamanickam T, Das J, et al. Topical anesthetic versus lidocaine infiltration in arteriovenous fistula cannulation. Chrismed Journal of Health and Research. 2014;**1**(2)

[130] Parisotto MT, Schoder VU, Miriunis C, Grassmann AH, Scatizzi LP, Kaufmann P, et al. Cannulation technique influences arteriovenous fistula and graft survival. Kidney International. 2014;**86**(4):790-797

[131] Ball LK. The buttonhole technique for arteriovenous fistula cannulation. Nephrology Nursing Journal. 2006;**33**(3):299-304

[132] Verhallen AM, Kooistra MP, van Jaarsveld BC. Cannulating in haemodialysis: Rope-ladder or buttonhole technique? Nephrology, Dialysis, Transplantation. 2007;**22**(9):2601-2604

[133] van Loon MM, Goovaerts T, Kessels AG, van der Sande FM, Tordoir JH. Buttonhole needling of haemodialysis arteriovenous fistulae results in less complications and interventions compared to the rope-ladder technique. Nephrology, Dialysis, Transplantation. 2010;**25**(1):225-230

[134] Macrae JM, Ahmed SB, Hemmelgarn BR, Alberta Kidney Disease N. Arteriovenous fistula survival and needling technique: Long-term results from a randomized buttonhole trial. American Journal of Kidney Diseases. 2014;**63**(4):636-642

[135] Parisotto MT, Pelliccia F, Furlan A, Pinto B, Miriunis C, Morris I, et al. Vascular Access Cannulation and Care: A Nursing Best Practice Guide for Arteriovenous Graft. 2nd ed. European Dialysis and Transplant Nurses Association/European Renal Care Association (EDTNA/ERCA); 2017

[136] Saran R, Dykstra DM, Wolfe RA, Gillespie B, Held PJ, Young EW. Association between vascular access failure and the use of specific drugs: The Dialysis Outcomes and Practice Patterns Study (DOPPS). American Journal of Kidney Diseases. 2002;**40**(6):1255-1263

[137] Sanada S, Miyasaka Y, Kanno A, Sato K, Sato M, Sugai H, et al. Efficacy of statin on vascular access patency in diabetic hemodialysis patients. The Journal of Vascular Access. 2017;**18**(4):295-300

[138] Righetti M, Ferrario G, Serbelloni P, Milani S, Tommasi A. Some old drugs improve late primary patency rate of native arteriovenous fistulas in hemodialysis patients. Annals of Vascular Surgery. 2009;**23**(4):491-497

[139] Chang H-H, Chang Y-K, Lu C-W, Huang C-T, Chien C-T, Hung K-Y, et al. Statins improve long term patency of arteriovenous fistula for hemodialysis. Scientific Reports. 2016;**6**:22197

[140] Tanner NC, Da Silva A. Medical adjuvant treatment to increase patency of arteriovenous fistulae and grafts. Cochrane Database of Systematic Reviews. 2015;7:CD002786

[141] Himmelfarb J, Couper L. Dipyridamole inhibits PDGF- and bFGF-induced vascular smooth muscle

cell proliferation. Kidney International. 1997;**52**(6):1671-1677

[142] da Silva OM, Rigon E, Dalazen JVC, Bissoloti A, Rabelo-Silva ER. Pain during arteriovenous fistula cannulation in chronic renal patients on hemodialysis. Open Journal of Nursing. 2016;**6**:1028-1037

[143] Besarab A, Kumbar L. Vascular access cannulation practices and outcomes. Kidney International. 2014;**86**(4):671-673

[144] Maria Teresa Parisotto Jitka Pancirova. Vascular Access: Cannulation and Care—A Nursing Best Practice Guide EDTA/ERCA. 2014

[145] Parisotto MT, Pelliccia F, Grassmann A, Marcelli D. Elements of dialysis nursing practice associated with successful cannulation: Result of an international survey. The Journal of Vascular Access. 2017;**18**(2):114-119

[146] WHO Guidelines Approved by the Guidelines Review Committee. WHO Guidelines on Hand Hygiene in Health Care: First Global Patient Safety Challenge Clean Care Is Safer Care. Geneva: World Health Organization; 2009

[147] Ullman AJ, Cooke ML, Mitchell M, Lin F, New K, Long DA, et al. Dressings and securement devices for central venous catheters (CVC). Cochrane Database of Systematic Reviews;(2015, 9):CD010367

[148] Porter ME, Teisberg EO. Redefining Health Care: Creating Value-Based Competition on Results. Boston: Harvard Business School Press; 2006

[149] Hu H, Patel S, Hanisch JJ, Santana JM, Hashimoto T, Bai H, et al. Future research directions to improve fistula maturation and reduce access failure. Seminars in Vascular Surgery. 2016;**29**(4):153-171

[150] Fraser SD, Roderick PJ, May CR, McIntyre N, McIntyre C, Fluck RJ, et al. The burden of comorbidity in people with chronic kidney disease stage 3: A cohort study. BMC Nephrology. 2015;**16**:193

[151] Work J. Hemodialysis catheters and ports. Seminars in Nephrology. 2002;**22**(3):211-220

[152] Konner K. History of vascular access for haemodialysis. Nephrology, Dialysis, Transplantation. 2005;**20**(12):2629-2635

[153] Whittier WL. Surveillance of hemodialysis vascular access. Semin Intervent Radiology. 2009;**26**(2):130-138

[154] Sato T, Tsuboi M, Onogi T, Miwa N, Sakurai H, Ookubo K, et al. Standard procedures of endovascular treatment for vascular access stenosis in our facility—Clinical usefulness of ultrasonography. The Journal of Vascular Access. 2015;**16**(Suppl 10): S34-S37

[155] Majerus S, Dunning J, Potkay JA, Bogie KM. Flexible, structured MWCNT/PDMS sensor for chronic vascular access monitoring. 2016 IEEE Sensors Conference. Orlando, FL: Oral presentation. 30 Oct-2 Nov, 2016

[156] Aragoncillo I, Abad S, Caldes S, Amezquita Y, Vega A, Cirugeda A, et al. Adding access blood flow surveillance reduces thrombosis and improves arteriovenous fistula patency: A randomized controlled trial. The Journal of Vascular Access. 2017;**18**(4):352-358

[157] Arechabala MC, Catoni MI, Claro JC, Rojas NP, Rubio ME, Calvo MA, et al. Antimicrobial lock solutions for preventing catheter-related infections in haemodialysis. Cochrane Database of Systematic Reviews. 2018;**4**:CD010597

[158] Rajan DK, Ebner A, Desai SB, Rios JM, Cohn WE. Percutaneous creation of an arteriovenous fistula for hemodialysis access. Journal of Vascular and Interventional Radiology. 2015;**26**(4):484-490

[159] Hull JE, Jennings WC, Cooper RI, Waheed U, Schaefer ME, Narayan R. The pivotal multicenter trial of ultrasound-guided percutaneous arteriovenous fistula creation for hemodialysis access. Journal of Vascular and Interventional Radiology. 2018;**29**(2):149-158. e5

[160] Collins MJ, Li X, Lv W, Yang C, Protack CD, Muto A, et al. Therapeutic strategies to combat neointimal hyperplasia in vascular grafts. Expert Review of Cardiovascular Therapy. 2012;**10**(5):635-647

[161] Pradhan-Nabzdyk L, Huang C, LoGerfo FW, Nabzdyk CS. Current siRNA targets in the prevention and treatment of intimal hyperplasia. Discovery Medicine. 2014;**18**(98):125-132

[162] Xu K, Al-Ani MK, Pan X, Chi Q, Dong N, Qiu X. Plant-derived products for treatment of vascular intima hyperplasia selectively inhibit vascular smooth muscle cell functions. Evidence-based Complementary and Alternative Medicine. 2018;**2018**:3549312

[163] Gage SM, Lawson JH. Bioengineered hemodialysis access grafts. The Journal of Vascular Access. 2017;**18**(Suppl 1):56-63

[164] Leermakers JJ, Bode AS, Vaidya A, van der Sande FM, Evers SM, Tordoir JH. Cost-effectiveness of vascular access for haemodialysis: Arteriovenous fistulas versus arteriovenous grafts. European Journal of Vascular and Endovascular Surgery. 2013;**45**(1):84-92

[165] Porter ME. What is value in health care? The New England Journal of Medicine. 2010;**363**(26):2477-2481

[166] Castellano I, Gallego S, Labrador PJ, Gomez-Martino JR, Covarsi A. The start of renal replacement therapy in a Spanish department. Nefrología. 2006;**26**(4):445-451

[167] Couchoud C, Moranne O, Frimat L, Labeeuw M, Allot V, Stengel B. Associations between comorbidities, treatment choice and outcome in the elderly with end-stage renal disease. Nephrology, Dialysis, Transplantation. 2007;**22**(11):3246-3254

[168] Chiu K, Alam A, Iqbal S. Predictors of suboptimal and crash initiation of dialysis at two tertiary care centers. Hemodialysis International. 2012;**16**(Suppl 1):S39-S46

[169] Nadeau-Fredette AC, Tennankore KK, Kim SJ, Chan CT. Suboptimal initiation of home hemodialysis: Determinants and clinical outcomes. Nephron Clinical Practice. 2013;**124**(1-2):132-140

[170] Hommel K, Madsen M, Kamper AL. The importance of early referral for the treatment of chronic kidney disease: A Danish nationwide cohort study. BMC Nephrology. 2012;**13**:108

[171] Canaud B, Tetta C, Marcelli D, Giordana G, Stuard S, Koehler K, et al. Implementation and Management of Strategies to Set and to Achieve Clinical Targets. Chapter 21. 2013. DOI: 10.5772/53041 [Accessed: January 24, 2019]

Section 2

Vascular Access and Reparative Surgery

Chapter 3

Endovascular Aortic Aneurysm Repair in Patients with Aortoiliac Occlusive Disease

Kevin D. Mangum, Arash Fereydooni and Naiem Nassiri

Abstract

Although endovascular aortic aneurysm repair (EVAR) has become an attractive, minimally invasive option for patients with abdominal aortic aneurysms (AAA), significant challenges in arterial access exist in patients with concomitant aortoiliac occlusive disease (AIOD), particularly for more advanced TASC C and D lesions. Under these circumstances, endograft delivery is possible but requires extensive preoperative planning and intraoperative techniques including but not limited to surgical conduit creation, plain balloon angioplasty, endoconduit placement, and subintimal recanalization. Newer generation aortic endografts have also shown promise in accommodating compromised access vessels. Concomitant AIOD and compromised access vessels complicate EVAR and increase operative time and complexity. Therefore, extreme caution, meticulous preoperative planning, familiarity and facility with the various surgical and endovascular options needed to circumvent these obstacles are essential for safe and effective delivery of EVAR in this high-risk subset of patients. The purpose of this chapter is to present standard approaches for access in patients undergoing EVAR; discuss how advanced AIOD precludes routine access; and present various methods to overcome difficult access in patients undergoing EVAR.

Keywords: abdominal aortic aneurysm, endovascular aortic aneurysm repair, aortoiliac occlusive disease, endograft, aorta, iliac artery, femoral artery, access, endoconduit

1. Introduction

Endovascular aortic aneurysm repair (EVAR) has expanded to more than 75% of elective abdominal aortic aneurysm (AAA) repairs due to its lower perioperative complication and high technical success rate [1, 2]. Despite its advantages, however, there are specific limitations that preclude EVAR delivery, making open AAA repair a more suitable option for select patients. In general, patient age and overall health are important considerations in deciding between EVAR versus open repair. Anatomic factors may also limit use of EVAR in select patients, and one of the single most important of these is proximal neck anatomy [3]. Unsuitable, hostile proximal neck features include angulation of ≥60°, neck length ≤ 10 mm, focal bulge in the neck >3 mm, and thrombus involving ≥50% of the aortic diameter—all common EVAR limiting factors [4]. In addition, access related issues due to atherosclerotic occlusive disease remain major barriers to EVAR as up to 36% of patients with AAA suffer from some degree of aortoiliac occlusive disease (AIOD) [5]. Concomitant AIOD may preclude EVAR in 6–15.4% of patients [6, 7]. The current Trans-Atlantic Inter-Society Consensus (TASC) guidelines consider an aneurysm in combination with a significant iliac artery stenosis or occlusion a TASC D lesion, and open surgical repair is suggested for these patients [8]. However, open repair is still associated with an in-hospital mortality rate of approximately 4%, particularly in this high-risk subset of patients with significant comorbidities that are associated with their peripheral arterial disease [9]. This combination of factors makes patients with AAA and AIOD even higher-risk candidates for open surgery.

Within the subset of patients with AAA and concomitant AIOD, about 15% require adjunctive access-related procedures to facilitate EVAR [10]. Furthermore, previously stented iliofemoral vessels are increasingly encountered and pose significant technical challenges for endovascular access and EVAR limb durability [11]. Overall, access-related complications—such as dissection and rupture—at the time of EVAR approach 10% compared to 15% in patients with concomitant AIOD [12]. Even though there has been a general reduction in device size in recent years compared with older generation aortic endoprostheses, some of the commonly used devices and most branched and fenestrated repair endovascular systems continue to require larger-diameter sheaths and delivery conduits. There are currently no clinical guidelines delineating the optimal therapy in patients with AAA and concomitant AIOD. Thus, familiarity with various techniques that can overcome compromised access vessels is essential for the modern-day vascular surgeon. These techniques have been developed to circumvent previously prohibitive anatomy and are discussed in this chapter. The emphasis herein will be on less invasive endovascular means of facilitating access in patients with compromised aortoiliac anatomy in the setting of AAA.

2. Access

2.1 Surgical access

The common femoral artery (CFA) is the most commonly accessed site for EVAR and has traditionally been approached via surgical cutdown. Typically, an incision is made parallel to and approximately two-finger breadths inferior to the inguinal ligament at the midway point between the anterior superior iliac spine and the pubic symphysis overlying the femoral pulse if palpable [13]. The superficial femoral fascia (contiguous with Scarpa's fascia) is divided obliquely, while the deep femoral fascia is divided parallel to femoral artery.

In cases of severely diseased or occluded CFAs, focal endarterectomy with patch angioplasty may be necessary prior to or immediately after EVAR to avoid limb-threatening ischemia and to facilitate EVAR delivery. Longitudinal skin incisions extending inferiorly from the inguinal ligament distally to the femoral bifurcation are preferred under these circumstances to facilitate adequate endarterectomy with profundaplasty if necessary. The proximal superficial femoral artery (SFA)—if patent and relatively disease-free—might be another option for access in cases of compromised CFAs or hostile groins. In such cases, the SFA is accessed via direct surgical cutdown along the medial border of the sartorius muscle [14].

2.2 Percutaneous access

Percutaneous access for EVAR was initially described in 1999, when the Prostar XL device (Abbot Vascular, Abbott Park, IL) was used for suture-mediated closure of femoral arteries [15]. The device is indicated for closure of vessels after percutaneous access of up to 10 Fr. If required, multiple devices can be used for larger caliber access closure [16].

The more popular Perclose ProGlide device (Abbot Vascular, Abbott Park, IL) is indicated for femoral access closure of up to 8 Fr for each closure device. It differs from the Prostar XL device in that it uses a single monofilament polypropylene suture instead of two braided polyester sutures. Multiple Perclose devices can be used to achieve closure for larger caliber arteriotomies up to 24 Fr inner diameter. This is achieved by deploying Perclose devices 45° clockwise and counterclockwise relative to the initially deployed device at the 12 o'clock position [17]. If needed, additional Perclose devices can be deployed for adequate hemostasis as long as wire access is maintained throughout the serial deployment process.

A recent meta-analysis of outcomes of percutaneous EVAR showed a technical success rate (defined as freedom from additional perioperative procedures) of 93%. There was an increased risk of conversion to cutdown when using sheaths ≥20 Fr [18]. Notably, both severe or anterior common femoral calcification and small access vessel diameter (<5 mm) have been associated with failed percutaneous access [18, 19]. In our own experience, we have found extreme iliac vessel tortuosity to be another predictor of unsuccessful percutaneous EVAR, given difficulty in closure device tracking and proper deployment of the footplate. To date, there has been no appropriately powered prospective, randomized study comparing percutaneous suture-mediated closure devices to open cutdown in EVAR. For now, a higher threshold for a total percutaneous approach and a readily available conversion mechanism to open surgical cutdown is advisable, particularly if one or more anatomically limiting factors are present.

3. Challenging access

3.1 Predicting access difficulty

In order to prevent inadvertent arterial injury and to avoid emergent measures, evaluation of the caliber and disease burden of all access vessels should be performed preoperatively based on adequate contrast-enhanced imaging. While computed tomography angiography (CTA) remains the preoperative imaging modality of choice, compromised access vessels may require catheter-directed angiography for pre-operative evaluation and/or treatment of access-related disease in anticipation of EVAR and for more appropriate device selection. The latter should be, in part, based on access vessel considerations such as patency, diameter, tortuosity, and severity of calcification. This is particularly important in older patients who have calcified, minimally elastic vessels and cannot tolerate excessive oversizing or stretching of the access vessels [20]. The minimum access vessel diameter requirement varies considerably based on the EVAR device manufacturer and the instructions for use (IFUs) for each particular device. A list of some of the commonly used endografts and their required iliac artery diameter has been provided in **Table 1**.

3.2 Conduit selection

Choice of conduit for EVAR delivery in the setting of AIOD is based on individual anatomy and disease severity. In general, TASC A and B disease may be amenable to simple balloon angioplasty of stenotic iliac arteries, after which the aortic endograft and/or required delivery sheath can be advanced. We caution against repeat balloon angioplasty and the use of oversized balloons due to associated life-threatening rupture that may result. In situations where simple angioplasty

Stent-graft	Graft diameter (mm)	Introducer sheath (F)	Access (outer) diameter (mm)
Abdominal aortic endograft			
Zenith Flex (Cook)	22–26	18	7.1
	28–32	20	7.7
	36	22	8.5
Excluder (Gore)	23–28	18	7.0
	31	20	7.6
Endurant II (Medtronic)	23–28	18*	7
	32–36	20*	7.6
AFX (Endologix)	22–28	17	6.5
Ovation (Endologix)	20–29	14	4.5
	34	15	4.5
Nellix (Endologix)	18–28	17	7
Thoracic aortic endograft			
Zenith Alpha (Cook)	24–30	16	6
	32–38	18	7.1
	40–44	20	7.7
TAG/C-TAG (Gore)	21	18	6.7
	26–28	20	7.5
	31–34	22	8.2
	37–45	24	8.8
Relay plus (Bolton)	22–32	22–23	8.3–8.7
	32–34	23–24	8.7–9.2
	36–40	24–25	9.2–9.3
	42	25	9.3
	44	25–26	9.3–9.5
	46	26	9.5
Valiant (Medtronic)	22–32	22*	8.3
	34–40	24*	9.2
	42–46	25*	9.3

Table 1.
*List of current abdominal and thoracic aortic endografts and their size specifications. *Represents outer diameter (OD) measurement (not sheath size) for Medtronic devices.*

does not seem to accommodate EVAR delivery, we recommend prophylactic covered stent placement prior to more aggressive angioplasty and the disruption of native vessel plaque. This technique provides a control mechanism if rupture occurs during angioplasty. For angioplasty alone, balloon diameter should not exceed the native vessel adventitia-to-adventitia diameter. Meticulous maintenance of guide wire access as well as immediately available balloon occlusion catheters and appropriately sized covered stents are strongly recommended at the time of angioplasty.

More advanced TASC C & D lesions often require a more comprehensive planning for safe and effective EVAR delivery. While open aortic surgery remains a consideration in these patients, high risk candidates warrant consideration for creative and less invasive endovascular approaches [21].

3.3 Surgical conduits

Open surgical conduits provide the advantage of larger conduits for device delivery and surgically exposed access for repair of any inadvertent arterial injury. Most surgical conduits are created at the distal common or proximal external iliac artery (EIA) using a lower retroperitoneal incision. The ideal strategy depends on the status of the iliac arteries (e.g., calcification and patency of internal iliac arteries) and the surgical risk for each individual patient. Most patients can tolerate a retroperitoneal exposure. However, this is a less ideal option in patients with hostile anatomy, prior surgery or radiation, retroperitoneal fibrosis, or in those with extensive comorbidities [20]. Standard surgical precautions should be taken to avoid ureteral injury and sympathetic plexus injury on the left side in men. Despite their advantages, however, surgical conduits should be used judiciously, given their reported association with longer operative times, hernias, prosthetic remnant infection, and prolonged recovery [22].

Although the common iliac artery (CIA) can be directly accessed with a sheath, a conduit often simplifies the procedure and provides increased availability of the iliac landing zone for EVAR. In creating the conduit, first the iliac arteries are controlled, and then a longitudinal arteriotomy is made anteriorly extending from the distal common to the external iliac artery [20]. A 10-mm Dacron graft is spatulated and anastomosed end-to-side to the native vessel. Of note, Fogarty occlusion balloon is a useful adjunct for vessel control in cases where severe calcification of the iliac arteries precludes safe and adequate surgical clamping [20].

A stab incision can be performed in the lower abdominal wall to exteriorize the conduit [23]. If there is severe external iliac occlusive disease, the conduit can be tunneled under the inguinal ligament to a counter incision in the groin to be converted to an iliofemoral bypass at the completion of the case [14]. This maneuver is also suitable for cases with planned repeat interventions in the future. Access is established via direct graft puncture after clamping and stabilizing the externalized distal end of the graft. Upon completion of the procedure, the conduit can be ligated and oversewn near the anastomosis leaving a short stump.

In cases with anticipated prolonged lower extremity ischemia time and patients with severe aortoiliac and profunda femoral disease, a temporary femoral artery conduit can be used to minimize lower extremity ischemia—reperfusion. A 10-mm femoral conduit is anastomosed end-to-side to the CFA using a standard oblique or longitudinal groin incision. The conduit allows periodic withdrawal of occlusive sheaths with restoration of flow while maintaining guide-wire access [20].

In cases with planned staged interventions for extensive thoracoabdominal repairs, permanent iliofemoral conduits are better options to avoid redo retroperitoneal exposure. Depending on patient anatomy and the extent of iliofemoral disease, there are several possible configurations. Iliofemoral bypass can be created from the distal CIA or proximal EIA to the proximal CFA, with access established into the graft after flow is restored to lower extremity [20].

Although direct iliac exposure might allow for better control of iliac injury, it is not without complications. In a study of 15,082 patients who underwent infrarenal EVAR from 2005 to 2012, 147 (1%) required iliac conduit or direct iliac access and had a higher rate of long-term mortality. [24] Compared to standard bilateral femoral exposure, surgical conduits also have a 1.8-fold increase in perioperative complications and a 1.5-day increase in length of hospital stay, but have no statistically significant difference in early mortality [25]. Furthermore, compared to percutaneous access, iliac exposure is associated with increased overall morbidity, operative time, intraoperative transfusion, and length of stay [14].

3.4 Alternative adjunctive techniques

Yano et al. reported that 50 of 390 patients (12%) undergoing EVAR required adjunctive maneuvers for endograft delivery [10]. Several adjunctive maneuvers have been proposed for patients with compromised and/or tortuous iliac arteries to facilitate EVAR [26]. Infrainguinal mobilization and "pull-down" of redundant external iliac arteries as well as lower abdominal manual compression during device advancement have been reported [20]. Alternatively, snared brachial-femoral wire access allows for a "body-floss" effect to stabilize the advancement of the delivery system through acutely angulated, redundant iliac arteries [27, 28]. For the brachial-femoral technique, it is useful to have an extended shaft brachial sheath to prevent the wire from transecting the subclavian-aortic junction or other angulated arterial segments [22].

Serial dilatation of the iliac artery with rigid dilators can be attempted, but application of excessive force should be avoided. Using this approach, an endovascular dilator set (Cook Medical, Bloomington, Indiana) consisting of dilators ranging from 14 to 26 Fr may be used to gradually dilate narrow, diseased iliac arteries [29]. Alternatively, a Solopath (Terumo, Somerset, NJ) balloon-expandable sheath can also be used in select cases where tortuosity and plaque is the main limiting factor [20]. The malleable design and hydrophilic coating of the sheath enable smooth tracking through narrowed vessels while the expandable balloon dilates stenosis [30].

3.5 Endoconduits

Increased morbidity with surgical conduits has led to the development of endovascular measures that facilitate EVAR in the setting of compromised access vessels [31]. Stents or stent-grafts are used to dilate atretic iliac arteries, correct any underlying occlusive disease, and/or over-dilate the artery beyond its baseline-limited caliber. First described in a series of five patients in 2001, this technique involved sewing a 6-mm expanded polytetrafluoroethylene graft to a stent and backloading the device into a 6F sheath [10]. The stent portion of the device was deployed across the internal iliac artery (IIA) and the prosthetic portion across the external iliac artery. The prosthetic portion was exteriorized through the femoral artery, and a noncompliant balloon was used to dilate the external iliac artery from within the graft.

Later in 2007, the "pave and crack" technique was introduced. Common and external iliac arteries were lined with 10-mm balloon expandable or self-expanding stents, and the stents were then dilated to 9–12 mm to create a controlled rupture [32]. In a similar technique, a 12-mm Excluder contralateral iliac limb (Gore, Flagstaff, AZ) was deployed from the common iliac extending into the proximal common femoral artery [33]. For this technique, it has been recommended to dilate the endoconduit to approximately 2 mm larger than the outer diameter of the intended endoprosthesis to allow for successful device delivery.

When planned and performed properly, endovascular conduits can be less invasive and have shorter procedural and recovery times compared to surgical conduits. Risks—such as stent dislodgement, coverage of internal iliac artery, and rupture—can be largely avoided with a measured, planned approach; appropriate device selection based on anatomic considerations; as well as familiarity with the nuances of the chosen EVAR device, its specific IFUs, and delivery apparatus. At times, a staged approach to endoconduit delivery—comprised of iliofemoral revascularization using covered stents with or without concomitant femoral endarterectomy followed by EVAR at a later date—may be necessary. The staged approach allows for stent incorporation, minimizing the risk of stent dislodgement, and development of collateral network in cases of intentional branch vessel occlusion. Furthermore, bifurcated unibody endografts or aorto-uni-iliac stent grafts may be chosen to overcome certain anatomic configurations; the former is particularly useful in the setting of a diseased, narrow distal aortic domain and may be the best option for avoidance of iliac limb occlusion.

Our covered stent of choice for endoconduit creation is the Viabahn stent-graft (Gore, Flagstaff, AZ). This technique was first described in 2009 using a 13 mm × 10 cm Viabahn dilated to 12 mm and an 8 mm × 5 cm Viabahn dilated to 8 mm [34, 35]. If the common iliac artery is larger than 13 mm, a tapered 16–12 mm Excluder iliac limb (Gore, Flagstaff, AZ) can be used [20]. More recently, the Gore VBX balloon-expandable covered stent system has been introduced [36]. The L configuration of this stent graft allows for post-dilation of up to 16-mm diameter. It has become our stent graft of choice for more aggressive post-dilation of compromised iliac arteries. In general, balloon expandable covered stents are used proximally in less mobile ostial locations, while flexible self-expanding covered stents are better choices distally in the external iliac arteries and more tortuous vessels due to their greater flexibility (**Figures 1** and **2**).

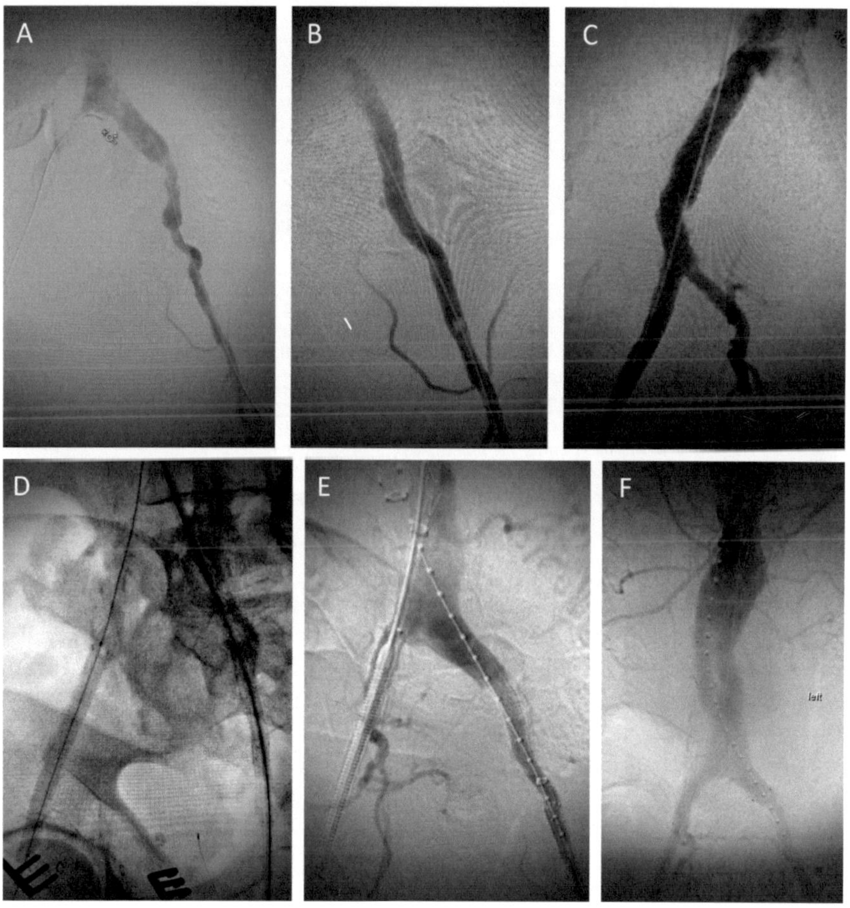

Figure 1.
(A) Diffusely diseased bilateral common and external iliac arteries precluding device advancement. (B, C) Endoconduits were created bilaterally with proximal VBX balloon expandable covered stents (Gore, Flagstaff, AZ), followed distally by self-expanding Viabahns (Gore, Flagstaff, AZ) extending into the proximal CFAs bilaterally. (C) Note the preserved patency of the right IIA. Post deployment angioplasty was performed with oversized balloons to facilitate easy (D) advancement and (E) deployment of an Endurant II aortic endograft (Medtronic, Minneapolis, Minnesota) and associated iliac limbs. (F) Completion angiogram demonstrated complete exclusion of the aneurysm sac without endoleak and unimpeded flow through the newly revascularized bilateral iliac arteries.

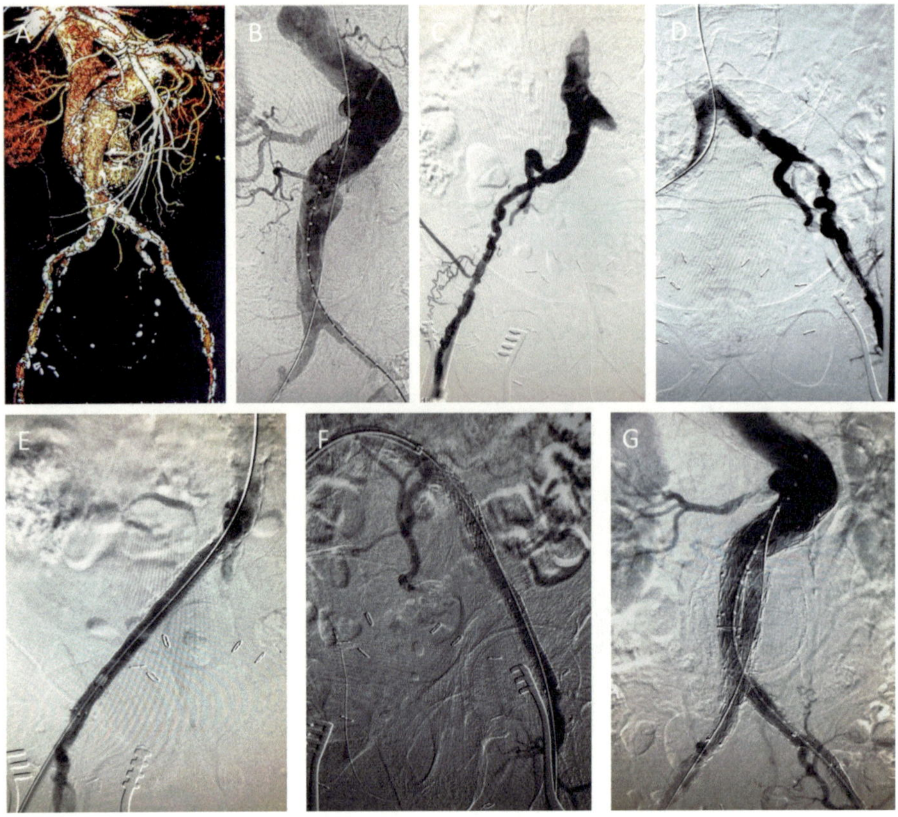

Figure 2.
(A) Three-dimensional reconstruction of the pre-operative CTA showing a juxtarenal abdominal aortic aneurysm with severe calcified stenosis of the bilateral common and external iliac arteries and occluded distal bilateral internal iliac arteries. (B) Flush abdominal aortography with bilateral iliofemoral runoff delineates shape and configuration of the aneurysm and confirms (C, D) the bilateral iliac disease burden. (E, F) Endoconduits were created using VBX balloon-expandable and Viabahn self-expanding covered stents (Gore, Flagstaff, AZ) bilaterally. The former are placed in the more proximal aspects of the diseased iliac arteries, while the latter are placed in the more mobile distal aspects of the iliac arteries to better accommodate hip flexion. Post-deployment angioplasty is an essential maneuver to ensure adequate endoconduit lumen diameter for advancing the device and to minimize risk of stent dislodgement during endograft delivery (G). Completion angiogram demonstrated complete exclusion of the AAA and a widely patent aortic endograft, CIAs, EIAs and left IIA without endoleak or kinks.

For advanced occlusive iliac lesions, covered stents are preferred over bare metal stents (BMS). The seminal COBEST study demonstrated that covered and BMS produced similar results for TASC B lesions; while for TASC C and D disease, covered stents had better long-term patency rates and lower reintervention rates [37]. Other advantages of covered stents over BMS include minimized in-stent neointimal hyperplasia and decreased risk of arterial perforation [38].

3.6 Angioplasty

Plain balloon angioplasty is favored as first-line strategy for low TASC-grade stenotic disease. We generally use 7–8-mm ultra-noncompliant balloons for passage of sheaths up to 18 Fr; 10-mm balloons for sheaths up to 22 Fr; and 12-mm balloons for 24 Fr sheaths.

When delivering devices that are not preloaded in sheaths, passage of the sheath dilator alone as the next step after ultra-noncompliant angioplasty of iliac occlusive disease is recommended [14]. The diameter of the dilator should be equal to or greater than the diameter of the anticipated endograft delivery mechanism.

Following this initial dilator passage step, the sheath and dilator are advanced together into the distal aorta. If the sheath meets obstruction, it is left in place, the dilator is removed, and the endograft is advanced "bareback" for the remaining length. Overdilating uncovered diseased or normal vessels to overcome a basic size mismatch is strongly discouraged due to risk of rupture. In such situations, endoconduits are better options, as they permit adequate angioplasty without risking iliac artery rupture in an uncontrolled fashion [10, 39]. When adequate distal and proximal seal is achieved via endoconduit creation, more aggressive angioplasty can be performed with lower risk for catastrophic hemorrhage [33].

3.7 Intraluminal or subintimal recanalization

Historically, in cases of severely diseased or occluded unilateral iliac arteries, aorto-uni-iliac stent-graft deployment with femoral-femoral bypass is performed [40, 41]. However, randomized trials have demonstrated approximately 20% lower long-term patency for femoral-femoral bypass compared to endovascular reconstruction in cases of unilateral iliac occlusive disease [42]. For EVAR, the aorto-uni-iliac configuration is also associated with inferior early and midterm outcomes as well as increased risk of graft infection [43, 44]. Therefore, in appropriately selected elective cases, intraluminal or subintimal recanalization from either brachial or femoral approach can be considered as alternative means of facilitating bifurcated EVAR device delivery [21]. Of note, successful subintimal recanalization has been described to facilitate bifurcated endograft placement in the presence of bilateral common iliac occlusive disease, making it an appropriate EVAR delivery method in select patients [14].

3.8 New generation of aortic endografts

The newest generation of ultra-low profile endografts allows for the treatment of AAAs in patients who were previously not candidates because of diseased and/or small access vessels. The Ovation Prime (Endologix, Irvine, California) stent graft system is delivered through a 14-Fr sheath. In the Ovation international pivotal trial, 40% of patients treated had access vessels smaller than 6 mm—the smallest access vessel was 4.7 mm in diameter—with a reported technical success rate of 100%; [45, 46]. Other low-profile devices currently in development or with limited approved use in the United States are the Incraft (Cordis Corp., Bridgewater, NJ) 13–15 Fr delivery system and the Zenith Low Profile (Cook Medical, Bloomington, IN) 16-Fr delivery system [47].

The AFX bifurcated unibody aortic endograft (Endologix, Irvine, California)—FDA-approved for EVAR—has also been successful in treating TASC D AIOD lesions with primary and assisted primary patency rates of 91 and 97% at 1 year, respectively (**Figure 3**) [48]. Unlike traditional modular bifurcated aortic endografts with fixation points at the infrarenal proximal aortic neck, the AFX is fixed at the aortic bifurcation [49]. Furthermore, it is delivered through a 17-Fr ipsilateral and a 9-Fr contralateral sheath facilitating advancement and deployment in heavily calcified, small-caliber iliac arteries [49]. In a recent study, the AFX unibody stent was successfully used in the treatment of TASC C/D lesions in patients with concomitant AAA [50]. At 1-year follow-up, no adverse events were reported; however, two patients required stenting of their EIAs due to worsening disease [50].

The Nellix Endovascular sealing system (Endologix, Irvine, California) is an investigational device that has a femoral access diameter requirement of at least 7-mm and involves injecting a biostable polyethylene glycol polymer into "endobags," which allow exclusion of the aneurysm and prevention of type 2 endoleaks

[51]. It has been successfully used in unilateral and bilateral common iliac artery occlusive disease ranging from 70% stenosis to complete occlusion [52]. In a study of Nellix system in five patients who had some degree of AIOD, occluded arteries were pretreated with balloon-expandable covered stents to create a patent conduit to accommodate the Nellix endograft. The aortic endograft was deployed successfully in 100% of cases without any endoleak at 9 months follow-up. Notably, this system has also been described in one case of infrarenal aortic stenosis, indicating that it has wider applicability in various degrees of AIOD [53, 54].

3.9 Common complications and management

The overall perioperative and long-term complication rates in patients with difficult EVAR access vessels have been reported to be 12 and 6%, respectively. Most commonly reported complication rates in the literature include 2.6–3.6% iliac rupture rates, 6% arterial dissections, 1.6–4% lower extremity ischemia, and 14% access site hematomas [10, 28, 41].

Iliac rupture from access is the leading cause of procedure-related mortality. If the guide wire is still in place, artery ruptures are better managed with endovascular placement of covered stents and usually do not require conversion to an open procedure. If a covered stent is not immediately available, an occlusive balloon catheter can be inserted and insufflated proximal to the rupture to achieve relative hemostasis without further damage at the rupture site until a stent graft or more definitive means of repair is delivered. In deploying covered stents for treatment of inadvertent arterial rupture, it is important to achieve long proximal and distal seal zones as the damage to the vessel is often more extensive than suggested by angiography [14]. A 10-cm self-expanding covered stent provides adequate proximal and distal seal in most cases. Iliac arteries less than 5-mm in diameter are considered to

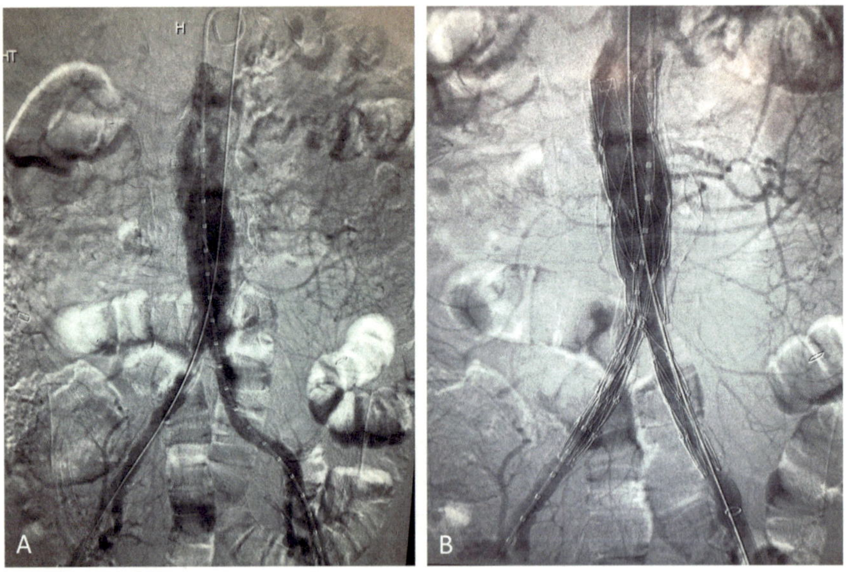

Figure 3.
(A) Intraoperative angiogram showing an infrarenal abdominal aortic aneurysm with concomitant severely symptomatic, nearly occlusive right proximal common iliac artery and high-grade stenosis of the proximal to mid-left common iliac artery. Note the diffusely diseased, narrow external iliac arteries along with a narrow distal aortic domain—all of which render deployment of a modular bifurcated device challenging and prone to complications including inadequate opening of the contralateral gate and iliac limb occlusions. (B) An AFX bifurcated unibody endograft (Endologix, Irvine, California) is preferred under these circumstances to treat both the AAA and the AIOD. Completion angiogram demonstrating complete exclusion of the AAA and a widely patent aortic endograft, CIAs, and EIAs without endoleak or kinks.

be more prone to rupture; therefore, prophylactic adjunctive procedures should be considered in these patients [41]. Almost all open iliac repairs are associated with postoperative morbidity [55].

The most feared complication is "iliac-artery-on-a-stick" or avulsion of the external iliac artery due to passage of a sheath in the setting of size mismatch. In most cases, the damage occurs initially with introduction of the sheath, but does not become obvious until the sheath is removed. This complication can be suspected when a large sheath suddenly advances easily after initial difficulty and can be avoided by proceeding with prophylactic endoconduit creation. If iliac avulsion is confirmed, an occlusion balloon may be left in place during sheath removal for immediate control. Conversion to open iliac artery exposure and endovascular reconstruction are both practical options. Proximally, the covered stent is bridged with stents to the aortic endograft. Hemorrhage from the internal iliac artery can be controlled with embolization or intentional ostial coverage. If adequate repair of rupture requires distal extension of the stent-graft well into the CFA, surgical modification and incorporation of the covered stent in to the common femoral artery is recommended.

In patients undergoing branched or fenestrated aortic endovascular repairs (FB-EVAR), hostile iliac anatomy due to calcification, stenosis, or tortuosity does not significantly affect the early outcome of FB-EVAR in terms of technical success and 30-day mortality. However, procedures performed in patients with such characteristics are technically more demanding and the adverse iliac anatomy is associated with reduced 3-year survival [56].

4. Conclusions

Patients with coexisting aortic aneurysms and aortoiliac occlusive disease represent a challenging subset at risk for higher perioperative and long-term complications rates following EVAR. Nevertheless, advancing endovascular stent graft technology and increased surgeon familiarity with prophylactic and bail-out techniques have increasingly facilitated EVAR in patients traditionally deemed unsuitable candidates given their compromised access vessels and iliac landing zones. Preoperative planning is essential for successful delivery of these multifaceted techniques that require a wide range of adjunctive equipment and preparatory maneuvers to prevent life-threatening complications. Next generation aortic stent grafts may forego the need for these adjunctive modalities via lower profile delivery means.

Conflict of interest

Nassiri: Consultant and Speakers' Bureau, W.L. Gore, INC.

Abbreviations

AAA	abdominal aortic aneurysm
AIOD	aortoiliac occlusive disease
BMS	bare metal stent
CFA	common femoral artery
CIA	common iliac artery
CTA	computed tomography angiography
EIA	external iliac artery
EVAR	endovascular aortic aneurysm repair

FB-EVAR	fenestrated-branched endovascular aortic aneurysm repair
Fr	French
IFU	instructions for use
IIA	internal iliac artery
SFA	superficial femoral artery
TASC	transatlantic inter-society consensus

Author details

Kevin D. Mangum[1], Arash Fereydooni[2] and Naiem Nassiri[3,4*]

1 University of North Carolina School of Medicine, Chapel Hill, NC,USA

2 School of Medicine, Yale University, New Haven, CT, USA

3 Department of Surgery, Division of Vascular & Endovascular Surgery, School of Medicine, Yale University, New Haven, CT, USA

4 VA Connecticut Healthcare System, West Haven, CT, USA

*Address all correspondence to: naiem.nassiri@yale.edu

References

[1] Lun Y et al. Comparison of midterm outcomes between surgical treatment and endovascular reconstruction for chronic infrarenal aortoiliac occlusion. Journal of Vascular and Interventional Radiology. 2015;**26**(2):196-204

[2] Schermerhorn ML et al. Changes in abdominal aortic aneurysm rupture and short-term mortality, 1995-2008: A retrospective observational study. Annals of Surgery. 2012;**256**(4):651-658

[3] Aburahma AF et al. Clinical outcomes for hostile versus favorable aortic neck anatomy in endovascular aortic aneurysm repair using modular devices. Journal of Vascular Surgery. 2011;**54**(1):13-21

[4] Dillavou ED et al. Does hostile neck anatomy preclude successful endovascular aortic aneurysm repair? Journal of Vascular Surgery. 2003;**38**(4):657-663

[5] Henretta JP et al. Special iliac artery considerations during aneurysm endografting. American Journal of Surgery. 1999;**178**(3):212-218

[6] Arko FR et al. How many patients with infrarenal aneurysms are candidates for endovascular repair? The Northern California experience. Journal of Endovascular Therapy. 2004;**11**(1):33-40

[7] Joels CS et al. Changing indications and outcomes for open abdominal aortic aneurysm repair since the advent of endovascular repair. The American Surgeon. 2009;**75**(8):665-669; discussion 669-70

[8] Norgren L et al. Inter-society consensus for the management of peripheral arterial disease (TASC II). Journal of Vascular Surgery. 2007;**45**(Suppl S):S5-S67

[9] Greenhalgh RM et al. Endovascular versus open repair of abdominal aortic aneurysm. The New England Journal of Medicine. 2010;**362**(20):1863-1871

[10] Yano OJ et al. Ancillary techniques to facilitate endovascular repair of aortic aneurysms. Journal of Vascular Surgery. 2001;**34**(1):69-75

[11] Daab LJ et al. Endovascular repair of an abdominal aortic aneurysm in a patient with stenosis of bilateral common iliac artery stents. Annals of Vascular Surgery. 2011;**25**(1):133.e9-133.e12

[12] Fairman RM et al. Pivotal results of the medtronic vascular talent thoracic stent graft system: The VALOR trial. Journal of Vascular Surgery. 2008;**48**(3):546-554

[13] Wind GG, Valentine RJ. Anatomic Exposures in Vascular Surgery, 2nd ed. Philadelphia: Lippincott Williams & Wilkins; 2013

[14] Minion DJ, Davenport DL. Access techniques for EVAR: Percutaneous techniques and working with small arteries. Seminars in Vascular Surgery. 2012;**25**(4):208-216

[15] Haas PC, Krajcer Z, Diethrich EB. Closure of large percutaneous access sites using the prostar xl percutaneous vascular surgery device. Journal of Endovascular Therapy. 1999;**6**(2):168-170

[16] Teh LG et al. Use of the percutaneous vascular surgery device for closure of femoral access sites during endovascular aneurysm repair: Lessons from our experience. European Journal of Vascular and Endovascular Surgery. 2001;**22**(5):418-423

[17] Dosluoglu HH et al. Total percutaneous endovascular repair of abdominal aortic aneurysms using

perclose proglide closure devices. Journal of Endovascular Therapy. 2007;**14**(2):184-188

[18] Eisenack M et al. Percutaneous endovascular aortic aneurysm repair: A prospective evaluation of safety, efficiency, and risk factors. Journal of Endovascular Therapy. 2009;**16**(6):708-713

[19] Traul DK et al. Percutaneous endovascular repair of infrarenal abdominal aortic aneurysms: A feasibility study. Journal of Vascular Surgery. 2000;**32**(4):770-776

[20] Baker AC, Oderich GS. Techniques of iliofemoral conduit for endovascular repair. In: Oderich GS, editor. Endovascular Aortic Repair: Current Techniques with Fenestrated, Branched and Parallel Stent-Grafts. Cham: Springer International Publishing; 2017. pp. 337-346

[21] Vallabhaneni R et al. Iliac artery recanalization of chronic occlusions to facilitate endovascular aneurysm repair. Journal of Vascular Surgery. 2012;**56**(6):1549-1554; discussion 1554

[22] Oderich GS, Picada-Correa M, Pereira AA. Open surgical and endovascular conduits for difficult access during endovascular aortic aneurysm repair. Annals of Vascular Surgery. 2012;**26**(7):1022-1029

[23] Criado FJ. Iliac arterial conduits for endovascular access: Technical considerations. Journal of Endovascular Therapy. 2007;**14**(3):347-351

[24] Nzara R et al. Perioperative outcomes in patients requiring iliac conduits or direct access for endovascular abdominal aortic aneurysm repair. Annals of Vascular Surgery. 2015;**29**(8):1548-1553

[25] Lee WA et al. Morbidity with retroperitoneal procedures during endovascular abdominal aortic aneurysm repair. Journal of Vascular Surgery. 2003;**38**(3):459-463; discussion 464-5

[26] Bischoff MS et al. Challenging access in endovascular repair of infrarenal aortic aneurysms. The Journal of Cardiovascular Surgery. 2014;**55** (2 Suppl 1):75-83

[27] Murray D et al. Access for endovascular aneurysm repair. Journal of Endovascular Therapy. 2006;**13**(6):754-761

[28] Fairman RM et al. Endovascular repair of aortic aneurysms: Critical events and adjunctive procedures. Journal of Vascular Surgery. 2001;**33**(6):1226-1232

[29] Bracale UM, Giribono AM, Spinelli D, Del Guercio L, Pipito N, Ferrara D, et al. Long-term results of endovascular treatment of TASC C and D aortoiliac occlusive disease with expanded polytetrafluoroethylene stent graft. Annals of vascular surgery. 2018

[30] Dimitriadis Z et al. Balloon expandable sheath for transfemoral aortic valve implantation: A viable option for patients with challenging access. Journal of Interventional Cardiology. 2013;**26**(1):84-89

[31] van Bogerijen GHW et al. Alternative access techniques with thoracic endovascular aortic repair, open iliac conduit versus endoconduit technique. Journal of Vascular Surgery. 2014;**60**(5):1168-1176

[32] Hinchliffe RJ et al. "Paving and cracking": An endovascular technique to facilitate the introduction of aortic stent-grafts through stenosed iliac arteries. Journal of Endovascular Therapy. 2007;**14**(5):630-633

[33] Peterson BG, Matsumura JS. Internal endoconduit: An innovative technique to address unfavorable

iliac artery anatomy encountered during thoracic endovascular aortic repair. Journal of Vascular Surgery. 2008;**47**(2):441-445

[34] Kpodonu J et al. "Cracking and paving": A novel technique to deliver a thoracic endograft despite ilio-femoral occlusive disease. Journal of Cardiac Surgery. 2009;**24**(2):188-190

[35] Wu T, Carson JG, Skelly CL. Use of internal endoconduits as an adjunct to endovascular aneurysm repair in the setting of challenging aortoiliac anatomy. Annals of Vascular Surgery. 2010;**24**(1):114.e7-114.e11

[36] Bismuth J et al. Pivotal study of a next-generation balloon-expandable stent-graft for treatment of iliac occlusive disease. Journal of Endovascular Therapy. 2017;**24**(5):629-637

[37] Mwipatayi BP et al. A comparison of covered vs bare expandable stents for the treatment of aortoiliac occlusive disease. Journal of Vascular Surgery. 2011;**54**(6):1561-1570

[38] Sabri SS et al. Outcomes of covered kissing stent placement compared with bare metal stent placement in the treatment of atherosclerotic occlusive disease at the aortic bifurcation. Journal of Vascular and Interventional Radiology. 2010;**21**(7):995-1003

[39] von Segesser LK et al. In situ introducer sheath dilatation for complex aortic access. European Journal of Cardio-Thoracic Surgery. 2002;**22**(2):316-318

[40] Makaroun MS. The Ancure endografting system: An update. Journal of Vascular Surgery. 2001;**33**(2, Part B): 129-134

[41] Etkin Y et al. Management of difficult access during endovascular aneurysm repair. Annals of Vascular Surgery. 2017;**44**:77-82

[42] Ricco JB, Probst H. Long-term results of a multicenter randomized study on direct versus crossover bypass for unilateral iliac artery occlusive disease. Journal of Vascular Surgery. 2008;**47**(1):45-54.e1

[43] O'Keeffe SD et al. Variations in early outcomes of endovascular aneurysm repair with alternate endograft configurations. Annals of Vascular Surgery. 2010;**24**(1):28-33

[44] Jean-Baptiste E et al. A comparison of the mid-term results following the use of bifurcated and aorto-uni-iliac devices in the treatment of abdominal aortic aneurysms. European Journal of Vascular and Endovascular Surgery. 2009;**38**(3):298-304

[45] Mehta M et al. One-year outcomes from an international study of the ovation abdominal stent graft system for endovascular aneurysm repair. Journal of Vascular Surgery. 2014;**59**(1):65-73. e1-3

[46] Nano G et al. Early experience with Ovation endograft system in abdominal aortic disease. Journal of Cardiothoracic Surgery. 2014;**9**:48-48

[47] Yassa E, Lombardi J. Infrarenal EVAR technology review. Endovascular Today. 2012;**11**:38-44

[48] Maldonado TS et al. Treatment of aortoiliac occlusive disease with the endologix AFX unibody endograft. European Journal of Vascular and Endovascular Surgery. 2016;**52**(1):64-74

[49] Kouvelos GN et al. Initial clinical experience with the endologix AFX unibody stent graft system for treating patients with abdominal aortic aneurysms: A case controlled comparative study. Vascular Specialist International. 2017;**33**(1):16-21

[50] Sirignano P et al. Results of AFX unibody stent-graft implantation in patients with TASC D aortoiliac lesions and coexistent abdominal aortic aneurysms. Journal of Endovascular Therapy. 2017;**24**(6):846-851

[51] Zoethout AC et al. Two-year outcomes of the Nellix endovascular aneurysm sealing system for treatment of abdominal aortic aneurysms. Journal of Endovascular Therapy : An Official Journal of the International Society of Endovascular Specialists. 2018;**25**(3):270-281

[52] van Sterkenburg SM et al. The Nellix endovascular sealing system in patients with abdominal aortic aneurysms in conjunction with iliac artery occlusive disease. Vascular. 2017;**25**(2):190-195

[53] Elbasty A, Crawford M, Morrow D. Endovascular aneurysm sealing for management of aortic occlusive disease. EJVES Short Reports. 2017;**37**:14-17

[54] Molnar RG, Gray WA. Sustained patency and clinical improvement following treatment of atherosclerotic iliac artery disease using the assurant cobalt iliac balloon-expandable stent system. Journal of Endovascular Therapy. 2013;**20**(1):94-103

[55] Duran C et al. A longitudinal view of improved management strategies and outcomes after iatrogenic iliac artery rupture during endovascular aneurysm repair. Annals of Vascular Surgery. 2013;**27**(1):1-7

[56] Gallitto E et al. Impact of iliac artery anatomy on the outcome of fenestrated and branched endovascular aortic repair. Journal of Vascular Surgery. 2017;**66**(6):1659-1667

Section 3

Vascular Access Failure

Chapter 4

Pathogenesis and Prevention of Vascular Access Failure

Rebecca Hudson, David Johnson and Andrea Viecelli

Abstract

Dialysis vascular access failure is common, is rated as a critical priority by both patients and health professionals, and is associated with excess morbidity, mortality and healthcare costs. This chapter will discuss the mechanisms underpinning vascular access failure as well as strategies for preventing this adverse outcome, including systemic medical therapies (such as antiplatelet agents, fish oils, statins, inhibitors of the renin-angiotensin-aldosterone system, and calcium channel blockers), and local therapeutic interventions including innovative surgical techniques, minimally invasive AVF creation, far infra-red therapy, perivascular application of recombinant elastase, endothelial loaded gel foam wrap (Vascugel), and antiproliferative agents such as sirolimus (Coll-R) and paclitaxel-coated balloon angioplasty.

Keywords: arteriovenous fistula, arteriovenous graft, arteriovenous shunt, aspirin, cardiovascular agents/therapeutic use, clinical research, endovascular procedures, end-stage kidney disease, fish oils, graft occlusion, hemodialysis, maturation, risk factors, statins, thrombosis, treatment outcome, vascular access, vascular patency

1. Introduction

The prevalence of end-stage kidney disease (ESKD) is increasing in the presence of a growing diabetic and aging population [1, 2]. Hemodialysis remains the most common form of kidney replacement therapy [3–5], with over 2 million people on hemodialysis worldwide [6]. To maintain successful hemodialysis, functional vascular access is required [7]. Hemodialysis vascular access consists of three forms: the arteriovenous fistula (AVF), the arteriovenous graft (AVG), and the central venous catheter (CVC). The AVF is a connection between a native artery and vein that is created via an end-to-side vein-to-artery anastomosis [8]. AVGs are created by interposing a prosthetic graft (classically with polytetrafluorethylene [PTFE]) between an artery and a vein [8]. The key requirements of such access are sufficient blood flow rate, low flow resistance, a low rate of complications and, for AVF and AVG, ease of cannulation.

A mature native AVF is considered superior to a synthetic AVG or CVC due to better long-term outcomes, including reduced rates of thrombosis, infection and interventions to maintain patency [9–11]. Balanced against these benefits, as a result of early thrombosis, neointimal hyperplasia formation and inadequate vasodilation (outward remodeling), between 20 and 60% of AVFs fail to mature to an adequate caliber to allow repeat cannulation and provide sufficient blood flow for hemodialysis and thereby prevent timely usability of the AVF for hemodialysis [9]. AVGs can be used within days of access creation but long-term, they are at higher risk of developing venous stenosis, thrombosis and infection compared to a functioning AVF [12]. More than 50% of AVGs thrombose within 12 months of creation and they require significantly more interventions to maintain patency compared to a functioning AVF [12–14]. CVCs can be used immediately after insertion, but their long-term use is discouraged in light of the significantly higher risks of thrombosis, catheter-associated bacteremia and inadequate solute clearance [15–17].

Vascular access dysfunction is a major cause of morbidity, mortality and excess healthcare costs [9, 18–20]. Indeed, healthcare professionals, patients and caregivers consider vascular access function a top priority of research in hemodialysis and clinical practice [21]. There have been recent advances in the understanding of the biology of vascular access and its dysfunction, with neointimal hyperplasia leading to venous stenosis and inadequate outward remodeling being identified as the two major causes of dialysis vascular access dysfunction [7, 22]. This knowledge has led to the identification of potential therapeutic targets and the development of novel interventions to improve and maintain vascular patency [17].

This chapter will discuss the risk factors for, and pathogenesis of arteriovenous access failure. The advances in the understanding of arteriovenous access failure have led to the development of therapeutic targets and novel therapeutic interventions including systemic medical therapies with pleiotropic effects (such as antiplatelet agents, fish oils, statins, inhibitors of the renin-angiotensin-aldosterone system [RAAS], and calcium channel blockers), and local therapeutic interventions including innovative surgical techniques, minimally invasive AVF creation, far infra-red therapy, perivascular application of recombinant elastase, endothelial loaded gel foam wrap (Vascugel), and antiproliferative agents such as sirolimus (Coll-R) and paclitaxel-coated balloon angioplasty.

2. Clinical predictors of arteriovenous access failure

Key contributors to successful AVF maturation and long-term function include adequate inflow properties determined by the size and quality of the feeding artery, cardiac output and blood pressure; anastomotic properties concerning the patent anastomosis between the artery and vein/interposition graft; and adequate outflow properties, which in turn are determined by the size and quality of the vein and presence or absence of collateral or accessory veins. The significance of these three factors in determining vascular access success highlight the importance of vascular mapping and planning prior to fistula creation.

Inflow properties are influenced by the location of the AVF, with patency increasing as the size of the feeding artery is increased (distal to proximal) [23]. Despite this, the distal radio cephalic AVF on the non-dominant side of the patient is the preferred initial site of AVF for vascular access [23], partly due to patient comfort along with the preservation of additional vascular access sites for future use. Female gender has been identified as a risk factor for failure of fistula maturation and survival, with investigations discovering significantly poorer outcomes of AVFs in females in comparison to males, though the reasons underpinning this are unclear [24–27]. It has been proposed that females have smaller vessels with associated decreased luminal diameters in comparison to males; however, this has not been consistently found to be a factor in unsuccessful AVFs [28, 29].

Key determinants of both inflow properties and anastomosis patency are the comorbidities of the patient undergoing AVF creation, influencing outcome via unfavorable effects on hemodynamics, with the most adverse effects seen from peripheral arterial disease, cardiovascular disease and diabetes mellitus. Peripheral arterial disease interferes with the remodeling process required to achieve a functioning fistula, involving the development of neointimal hyperplasia and calcification, causing increased arterial stiffness and decreased elasticity [30]. Woods et al. [31] conducted a study involving 784 incident hemodialysis patients and found a 24% increased risk of AVF failure in those with peripheral arterial disease. This failure is attributable to the fact that for vascular access to be a success, it is essential that the artery used in the creation of the fistula is able to adequately increase diameter allowing for the increased blood flow required to supply the fistula and distal tissues [32, 33].

In relation to cardiac disease, its adverse impact on fistula maturation is due to poor cardiac output and associated poor blood flow to the fistula, resulting in worse outcomes [34].

Diabetes mellitus is associated with increased risks of intimal hyperplasia [35], and peripheral arterial disease [36], with these risks exaggerated further in the chronic kidney disease population leading to an appreciable rate of AVF failure in this group [27, 37, 38].

Advancing age has been cited as a risk factor for failure of AVF maturation and survival, although this proves difficult to quantify with age also being a surrogate marker for increasing burden of comorbidities. Studies have indicated an increased failure rate of AVFs in 'older patients' with the definition of those greater than or equal to 65 years of age [39–41], contrasting with other literature which were unable to identify significant differences in functional access outcomes for older patients [26, 42].

Race and ethnicity have also been identified as risk factors for failure of AVF maturation, though again this has not been consistently replicated in the literature [43]. Studies however have identified AVF failure rate being more common in those of African racial background in comparison to Caucasians; along with Hispanics when compared with non-Hispanics [40, 41, 44].

A pertinent factor affecting the anastomosis and therefore the outcomes of AVFs includes both the experience of the surgeon in creating the fistula, as well as the technical issues associated with utilizing and managing the fistula. The formation of AVFs is difficult, with numerous studies indicating that there is a higher incidence of successful AVFs if the surgery is performed by an experienced vascular surgeon [45–49], with the emphasis being placed on the number of AVFs created over the total years of training [48, 50].

Outflow dynamics are influenced by several factors, one of which is obesity. Obesity is described as a risk factor for failure of vascular access separate to the increased incidence of diabetes in this group. It was observed that obese patients experienced poor secondary patency in a study by Kats et al. [51], with the underlying theory that this was due to the increased soft tissue mass leading to venous compression and outflow tract obstruction [52]. Diabetes has also been shown to be a negative predictor of venous remodeling [53], directly impacting the outflow from an AVF.

Following arteriovenous access creation, ongoing access surveillance, care and cannulation by well trained staff/patient are paramount for preventing access failure [54–59].

3. Pathophysiology of arteriovenous access dysfunction

The pathogenesis of vascular access failure is complex with the common final pathway being the combination of insufficient vessel vasodilation, negative (inward) vascular remodeling and neointimal hyperplasia resulting in luminal narrowing and often associated thrombosis formation. The Achilles heel of this process is the graft-vein anastomosis in AVG and the perianastomotic region in AVF, respectively [1, 13]. The pathophysiologic cascade of events that lead to AVF and AVG failure [16, 17] have been categorized into upstream events, characterized by factors that lead to injury of endothelial—and smooth muscle cells and downstream events describing the cellular and cytokine responses that leads to neointimal hyperplasia and inward remodeling [16] (**Figure 1**).

There are multiple factors that contribute to the upstream events of vascular access dysfunction: (1) the proinflammatory uremic milieu that promotes endothelial dysfunction [16, 60], (2) hemodynamic stressors at the anastomosis site due to a combination of small and non-compliant vessels, low shear stress and turbulence [16, 61, 62], (3) vascular injury at the time of fistula or graft formation due to vessel manipulation through surgical technique or angioplasty [16, 61, 62], (4) a localized inflammatory response involving cytokine release and macrophage migration caused by the synthetic graft material used in the formation of the AVG [16], (5) possible genetic predisposition to neointimal hyperplasia and vasoconstriction [11, 16] (6) and repeat cannulation injury [16, 54].

After formation of an AVF, rapid increase in blood flow through the feeding artery and draining vein causes vascular distension [63] leading to nitric oxide (NO) synthesis by endothelial cells which results in vascular smooth muscle relaxation and vasodilatation [64]. This response leads to structured vascular remodeling with the driving forces of wall shear stress and tension [63] leading to an increase in arterial and venous lumen size [65] and moderate thickening of the venous wall assisting in maturation [66] and positive (outward) remodeling, which overall results in a larger lumen and greater vascular success (**Figure 2**). In comparison, the smooth muscle and endothelial injury sustained from the upstream events described previously, trigger a cascade of downstream responses mediated through proinflammatory leukotrienes, chemokines, cytokines, vasoactive molecules, metalloproteinase and adhesion molecules that promote neointimal hyperplasia

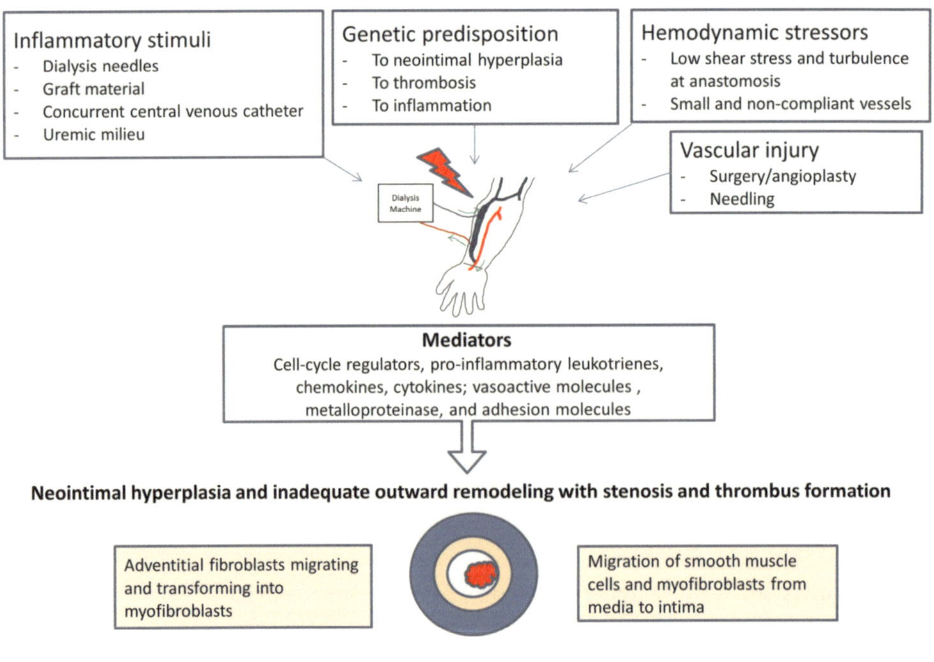

Figure 1.
Pathogenesis of vascular access failure. This figure illustrates the different pathogenic mechanisms that result in vascular access failure. Image re-used from Viecelli et al. [13] with permission from Wiley.

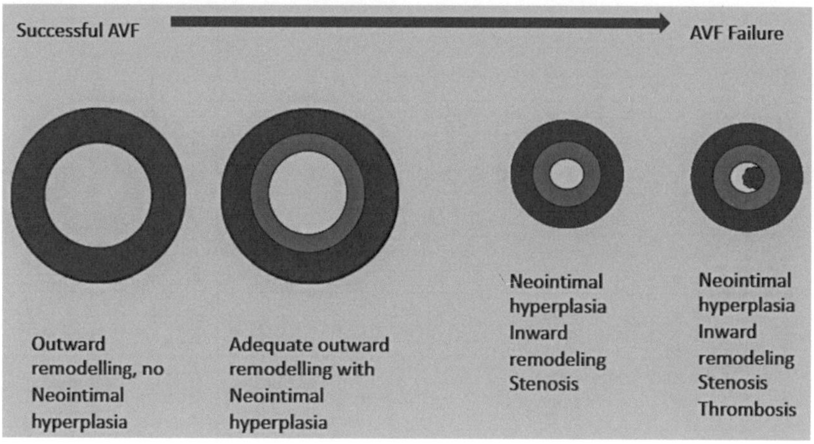

Figure 2.
Vascular remodeling response post fistula creation: comparison of the effects of neointimal hyperplasia with outward and inward vascular remodeling.

formation and negative (inward) remodeling. In comparison to outward remodeling, inward remodeling results in small lumen diameter and an increased risk of access failure [17]. As such, neointimal hyperplasia if combined with compensatory outward remodeling may not result in flow limiting stenosis due to preservation of the luminal caliber, whereas neointimal hyperplasia combined with impaired outward remodeling can result in hemodynamically significant vascular stenosis and resultant thrombosis [17, 63].

4. Therapeutic interventions to prevent VA dysfunction

The following section will discuss systemic medical and local interventions developed to minimize luminal narrowing caused by neointimal hyperplasia and negative (inward) vascular remodeling.

4.1 Systemic medical therapies

4.1.1 Antiplatelet agents

Antiplatelet agents including aspirin, dipyridamole, clopidogrel and ticlopidine are thought to prevent arteriovenous access failure primarily through their antithrombotic effect. Clinical trial results will be discussed separately for each agent given the differences in action of individual agents upon platelet aggregation, function and vascular biology including anti-inflammatory and antiproliferative properties.

4.1.1.1 Aspirin

Aspirin irreversibly inhibits platelet cyclooxygenase-1 and -2 enzymes via acetylation, resulting in decreased formation of prostaglandin precursors and prostaglandin derivative thromboxane A2 [13]. Randomized controlled trials (RCT) on the efficacy of aspirin in preventing arteriovenous access failure have shown inconsistent results, with two small studies favoring aspirin [67, 68] and two studies showing no significant treatment benefit for the prevention of arteriovenous access thrombosis and failure (**Table 1**) [5, 69]. In a small RCT of 44 patients, AVG thrombosis was significantly reduced with 160 mg of aspirin daily compared to

Trial	Study	Number of participants	Co-morbidities	Access type	Intervention	Control	Treatment duration (months)	Primary outcome (aspirin vs placebo)	Secondary outcome (aspirin vs placebo)
Aspirin									
Irish et al. [5].	RCT	388	HTN (94%), smoking history (54%), DM (49%), CAD (11%), PVD (4%), CHD (4%), CVD (3%)	AVF	Aspirin 100 mg daily	Placebo	3	Proportion of subjects with AVF failure (thrombosis, abandonment or cannulation failure) at 12 months *45% vs 47%, RR 1.05, 95% CI 0.84–1.31, p = 0.68*	AVF thrombosis at 12 months *20% vs 18%, RR 1.09, 95% CI 0.72–1.64, p = 0.70* AVF abandonment at 12 months *24% vs 18%, RR 1.31, 95% CI 0.89–1.95. p = 0.17* Cannulation failure at 12 months *40% vs 39%, RR 0.99, 95% CI 0.76–1.27, p = 0.92*
Harter et al. [67]	RCT	44	NR	AVG	Aspirin 160 mg daily	Placebo	4	Thrombosis at study end (mean 5 months) *32% vs 72%, OR o.18, 95% CI 0.05–0.66, p < 0.01*	Number of thrombotic events per patient month *0.16 vs 0.46, p < 0.05*
Andrassy et al. [68]	RCT	92	NR	AVF	Aspirin 1000 mg alternate days	Placebo	1	Thrombosis at 28 days *4% vs 23%, p < 0.05*	NR

Dipyridamole and/or aspirin

Trial	Study	Number of participants	Co-morbidities	Access type	Intervention	Control	Treatment duration (months)	Primary outcome (antiplatelet agent(s) vs placebo)	Secondary outcome (antiplatelet agent(s) vs placebo)
Sreedhara et al. [69]	RCT	107 (84 type I [new AVG] and 23	NR	AVG	Aspirin 325 mg daily, or Dipyridamole 225 mg + Aspirin	Placebo	18	Thrombosis at 18 months **Aspirin**—type I 50% vs	RR of thrombosis with new AVG Aspirin 1.99, 95% CI

Trial	Study	Number of participants	Co-morbidities	Access type	Intervention	Control	Treatment duration (months)	Primary outcome	Secondary outcome
		type II [thrombosed AVG requiring new AVG])			325 mg daily or Dipyridamole 225 mg daily			32%, type II 50% vs 80% **Aspirin + Dipyridamole**—type I 23% vs 32%, type II 100% vs 80% **Dipyridamole**—type I 17% vs 32%, type II 83% vs 80%	0.88–4.48, p = 0.18 Dipyridamole 0.35, 95% CI 0.15–0.80, p = 0.02
Clopidogrel									
Trial	**Study**	**Number of participants**	**Co-morbidities**	**Access type**	**Intervention**	**Control**	**Treatment duration (months)**	**Primary outcome (clopidogrel vs placebo)**	**Secondary outcome (clopidogrel vs placebo)**
Ghorbani et al. [73]	RCT	93	DM (26.9%)	AVF	Clopidogrel 75 mg daily	Placebo	1.5	Primary AVF failure at 8 weeks *5.2% vs 21.6%; HR 0.72, 95% CI 0.41–1.01, p = 0.03*	Successful HD within 6 months of AVF creation *92% vs 71%, p = 0.008*
Dember et al. [15]	RCT	877	Smoking history (62%), DM (48%), CAD (28%), CVD (6%), PVD (3%)	AVF	Clopidogrel 300 mg loading dose followed by 75 mg daily	Placebo	1.5	Thrombosis at 6 weeks post fistula creation *12% vs 20%, RR 0.63, 95% CI 0.46–0.97, p = 0.018*	Failure to attain suitability for dialysis *62% vs 60%, RR 1.05, 95% CI 0.94–1.17, p = 0.40*
Clopidogrel and aspirin									
Trial	**Study**	**Number of participants**	**Co-morbidities**	**Access type**	**Intervention**	**Control**	**Treatment duration (months)**	**Primary outcome (antiplatelet agents vs placebo)**	**Secondary outcome (antiplatelet agents vs placebo)**
Kaufman et al. [74]	RCT	200	DM (47%)	AVG	Aspirin 325 mg daily + Clopidogrel 75 mg daily	Placebo	NR	Cumulative incidence of thrombosis *HR 0.81, 95% CI 0.47–1.40, p = 0.45*	Cumulative incidence of first graft thrombosis for patients with grafts without previous thrombosis (n = 111) *HR 0.52, 95% CI 0.22–1.26, p = 0.14*

Ticlopidine

Trial	Study	Number of participants	Co-morbidities	Access type	Intervention	Control	Treatment duration (months)	Primary outcome (ticlopidine vs placebo)	Secondary outcome (ticlopidine vs placebo)
Grontoft et al. [77]	RCT	250	DM (27%)	AVF	Ticlopidine 250 mg twice daily	Placebo	1	Thrombosis at 4 weeks *12% vs 19%, OR 0.6, 95% CI 0.30–1.18, $p = 0.1$*	NR
Grontoft et al. [75]	RCT	36	DM (61%)	AVF	Ticlopidine 250 mg twice daily	Placebo	1	Thrombosis at 4 weeks *11% vs 47%, $p < 0.05$*	NR
Fickerstrand et al. [76]	RCT	18	NR	AVF	Ticlopidine 250 mg twice daily	Placebo	1	Thrombosis at 4 weeks *25% vs 50%*	NR

Omega-3 fatty acid supplementation (fish oil)

Trial	Study	Number of participants	Co-morbidities	Access type	Intervention	Control	Treatment duration (months)	Primary outcome (fish oil vs placebo)	Secondary outcome (fish oil vs placebo)
Irish et al. [5]	RCT	536	HTN (94%), smoking history (54%), DM (49%), CAD (11%), PVD (4%), CHD (4%), CVD (3%)	AVF	4 g of fish oil daily	Placebo	3	AVF failure (thrombosis, abandonment or cannulation failure) at 12 months *47% both groups, RR 1.03, 95% CI 0.86–1.23, $p = 0.78$*	AVF thrombosis at 12 months *22% vs 23%, RR 0.98, 95% CI 0.72–1.34, $p = 0.9$* AVF abandonment at 12 months *19% vs 22%, RR 0.87, 95% CI 0.62–1.2, $p = 0.43$* Cannulation failure at 12 months *40% vs 39%, RR 1.03, 95% CI 0.83–1.26, $p = 0.81$*
Lok et al. [89]	RCT	196	HTN (86%), smoking history (55%), DM	AVG	4 g of fish oil daily	Placebo	12	Proportion of participants	Rate of loss of graft patency

			(53%), CAD (33%), CHD (20%), PVD (15%), CVD (14%)					experiencing graft patency loss (thrombosis or radiological or surgical interventions) at 12 months *48% vs 62%, RR 0.78, 95% CI 0.60–1.03, p = 0.06*	*IRR 0.58, 95% CI 0.44–0.75* Radiological or surgical intervention to maintain patency *IRR 0.59, 95% CI 0.44–0.78* Thrombotic events *IRR 0.5, 95% CI 0.35–0.72*
Bowden et al. [90]	RCT	29	DM (69%), smoking history (3%)	AVG	6 g of fish oil daily	Placebo	8	Primary patency loss (thrombosis or venous outflow stenosis >50% requiring angioplasty) *254 ± 52 days, SEM 51.8 vs 254 ± 35 days, SEM 34.6, NS*	NR
Schmitz et al. [88]	RCT	24	DM (58%)	AVG	4 g of fish oil daily	Placebo	12	Primary patency (thrombosis free) at 12 months *75.6% vs 14.9%, p = 0.03*	NR
Statin therapy									
Trial	**Study**	**Number of participants**	**Co-morbidities**	**Access type**	**Intervention**	**Control**	**Treatment follow-up (years)**	**Primary outcome (statin vs placebo)**	**Secondary outcome (statin vs placebo)**
Herrington et al. [94]	Post hoc analysis of RCT	2353	DM (22%), smoking history (15%)	AVF (94%), AVG (6%)	Simvastatin (20 mg) plus Ezetimibe (10 mg) daily	Placebo	5	Vascular access occlusive event (access requiring any revision procedure, access thrombosis, removal of an old dialysis access, or formation of new permanent dialysis access)	Access revision 18.6% vs 21.4% RR 0.85, CI 0.67–1.08 Access thrombosis 9.3% vs 10.3% RR 0.90, CI 0.64–1.27 Removal of old or formation of new vascular access

								29.7 vs 33.5% RR 0.87, 95% CI 0.75–1.00, p = 0.05	15% vs 16.2% RR 0.93, CI 0.75–1.00
Herrington et al. [94]	Post-hoc analysis of RCT	2439	DM (27%), smoking history (14%)	AVF (89%), AVG (11%)	Rosuvastatin 10 mg daily	Placebo	4.5	Vascular access occlusive event 28.9% vs 27.6% RR 1.06, 95% CI 0.91–1.23, p = 0.44	NR
Birch et al. [91]	Retrospective analysis	265	HTN (93%), DM (53%)	AVF	Statin therapy of variable doses (Simvastatin, Atorvastatin, Pravastatin, Lovastatin)	No statin therapy	1.8	Interval of time to angioplasty to maintain AVF function *Mean time 8.9 vs 7.3 months, p = 0.25* Number of stenotic lesions *98 vs 99 stenoses, p = 0.28*	Primary AVF patency (time from creation to first intervention) *HR 1.17, 95% CI 0.747–1.834, p = 0.49*
Pisoni et al. [97]	Retrospective observational cohort analysis	601	HTN (92%), DM (52%), CAD (29%), PVD (18%), CVD (10%)	AVF (53%), AVG (47%)	Statin therapy not specified	No statin therapy	6	Primary access failure (access never useable for dialysis) **AVF** *37% vs 38%, OR 0.97, 95% CI 0.59–1.58, p = 0.9* **AVG** *20% vs 14%, OR 1.52, 95% CI 0.76–3.09, p = 0.23* Cumulative access survival **AVF** *HR 1.26, 95% CI 0.76–2.16, p = 0.35* **AVG** *HR 0.88, 95% CI 0.59–1.32, p = 0.54*	NR
Righetti et al. [34]	Case-control study	60	HTN, dyslipidemia	AVF	Atorvastatin 10–20 mg or Simvastatin 10–20 mg daily and/or folic acid 5 mg daily	No statin or folic acid therapy	3	Primary access patency *71.5% vs 39.1% after 2 years, p < 0.05*	NR

Saran et al. [96]	Retrospective observational cohort analysis	2462	HTN (87.8%), DM (49.7%), Obesity (35.9%)	AVF 900 (8.3% on statin), AVG 1944 (9.6% on statin)	Statin therapy of varying doses (Simvastatin, Atorvastatin, Pravastatin, Lovastatin) Fluvastatin)	NR	4	Primary access patency (unassisted access patency) ***AVG*** *RR 0.97, p = 0.805* ***AVF*** *RR 0.93, p = 0.762* Secondary access patency (assisted access survival) ***AVG*** *RR 1.01, p = 0.920* ***AVF*** *RR 1.03, p = 0.903*	NR

Renin-angiotensin-aldosterone system blockers (angiotensin-converting enzyme inhibitors and angiotensin II type I receptor blockers) therapy

Trial	Study	Number of participants	Co-morbidities	Access type	Intervention	Control	Treatment follow-up (years)	Primary outcome (ACEI/ARB vs placebo)	Secondary outcome
Chen et al. [108]	Retrospective analysis	42,244	HTN (81%), DM (51%), CAD (24%), Dyslipidemia (17%), CVD (6%), PVD (3%)	AVF 89.4% (32.3% on an ACEI, 15% on an ARB) AVG 10.6% (6.2% on an ACEI, 7.1% on an ARB)	ACEI/ARB therapy of varying doses **ACEI** (Benazepril, Enalapril, Lisinopril, Quinapril, Captopril, Fosinopril, Ramipril, Cilazapril) **ARB** (Candesartan, Losartan, Irbesartan, Valsartan, Olmesartan)	Non-use	8	Primary patency loss **AVF** *ACEI-HR 0.59, 95% CI 0.56–0.62, p < 0.05* *ARB-HR 0.53, 95% CI 0.51–0.56, p < 0.05* **AVG** *ACEI-HR 0.56, 95% CI 0.48–0.64, p < 0.05* *ARB-HR 0.54, 95% CI 0.47–0.61, p < 0.05*	NR
Jackson et al. [99]	Retrospective cohort analysis	332	DM (75%), HTN (62%), smoking history (36%)	AVF (64%) AVG (36%)	ARB therapy of varying doses (Irbesartan, Losartan, Valsartan)	Non-use	4	Primary patency loss **AVF** *HR 0.35, 95% CI 0.16–0.76, p = 0.008* **AVG** *HR 0.41, 95% CI 0.18–0.95, p = 0.04*	NR

Saran et al. [96]	Retrospective analysis	2462	HTN (87.8%), DM (49.7%), Obesity (35.9%)	AVF 900 (18.7% on ACEI, 4.1% on ARB), AVG 1944 (17% on ACEI, 3.8% on ARB)	ACEI/ARB therapy of varying doses **ACEI** (Benazepril, Enalapril, Lisinopril, Quinapril, Captopril, Fosinopril, Moexipril, Ramipril) **ARB** (Candesartan, Losartan, Irbesartan, Valsartan)	Non-use	4	**AVF** Unassisted primary access patency *ACEI-RR 0.77, $p = 0.09$* *ARB-RR 1.45, $p = 0.06$* Secondary access patency *ACEI-RR 0.56, $p = 0.01$* *ARB-RR 1.33, $p = 0.31$* **AVG** Primary access patency *ACEI-RR 1.02, $p = 0.85$* *ARB-RR 1.09, $p = 0.63$* Secondary access patency *ACEI-RR 1.16, $p = 0.13$* *ARB-RR 1.3, $p = 0.17$*	NR
Sajgure et al. [98]	Multicentre observational study	266	HTN (95%), DM (57%)	AVF (33%) AVG (67%)	ACEI of varying doses	Placebo	2	Primary patency duration (mean ± SEM) in days **AVG** *672 ± 68 vs 460 ± 48, HR 0.48, 95% CI 0.31–0.73, $p = 0.01$* **AVF** *530 ± 80 vs 501 ± 76, $p = 0.45$*	NR

Calcium channel blocker therapy

Trial	Study	Number of participants	Co-morbidities	Access type	Intervention	Control	Treatment follow-up (months)	Primary outcome	Secondary outcome
Saran et al. [96]	Retrospective observational	2462	HTN (87.8%), DM (49.7%), Obesity (35.9%)	AVF 900 (44.1% on CCB), AVG	CCB therapy of varying doses (Amlodipine,	Non-use	4	Unassisted primary access patency ***AVG*** *RR 0.86, $p = 0.034$*	NR

DOI: http://dx.doi.org/10.5772/intechopen.83525

	cohort analysis			1944 (40.8% on CCB)	Felodipine, Mibefradil, Nifedipine, Verapamil, Diltiazem, Isradipine, Nicardipine, Nisoldipine)			***AVF*** *RR 1.14, p = 0.3* Secondary access patency ***AVG*** *RR 0.88, p = 0.153* ***AVF*** *RR 1.16, p = 0.374*	
Chen et al. [108]	Retrospective analysis	42,244	HTN (81%), DM (51%), CAD (24%), Dyslipidemia (17%), CVD (6%), PVD (3%)	AVF 89.4% (32.3% on CCB), AVG 10.6% (20.6% on CCB)	CCB therapy of varying doses (Amlodipine, Felodipine, Nifedipine, Verapamil, Diltiazem, Isradipine, Nicardipine)	Non-use	8	Primary patency loss ***AVF*** *HR 0.485, CI 0.470–0.501* ***AVG*** *HR 0.482, CI 0.442–0.526*	NR

New surgical techniques to optimize flow dynamics

Trial	Study	Number of participants	Co-morbidities	Access type	Intervention	Control	Treatment follow-up (months)	Primary outcome	Secondary outcome
Chemla et al. [127]	Prospective study	41	NR	AVF	Optiflow device	NR	3	Unassisted maturation (outflow vein >/= 5 mm in diameter and flow >/= 500 ml/min not requiring intervention to maintain or promote maturation) *72% at 42 days & 68% at 90 days* Unassisted patency *88% at 42 days & 78% at 90 days*	NR
Bharat et al. [126]	Comparative study	125	HTN (43%), DM (41%)	AVF	pSLOT vs SLOT vs ETS	NR	19	Formation of juxta-anastomotic stenosis *pSLOT (3.7%, p = 0.04) vs SLOT (8.3%, p = NS) vs ETS (14%, p = NS)* Fistula failure	NR

								(pSLOT 16.7%, $p = 0.01$), SLOT (33.3%, p = NS), ETS (40.3%, p = NS)	
Endovascular AVF creation									
Trial	**Study**	**Number of participants**	**Co-morbidities**	**Access type**	**Intervention**	**Control**	**Treatment follow-up (months)**	**Primary outcome**	**Secondary outcome**
Lok et al. [114]	Prospective study	80	HTN (92%), DM (65%), CAD (22%), CVD (15%), CHD (12%), PVD (5%)	AVF	Endovascular AVF creation	NR	12	Percentage of endovascular AVF suitable for HD at 3 months *91%, 95% CI 81–97%*	Primary patency at 12 months *69%, 95% CI 54–79%* Cumulative patency at 12 months *84%, 95% CI 71–91%*
Far infrared therapy									
Trial	**Study**	**Number of participants**	**Co-morbidities**	**Access type**	**Intervention**	**Control**	**Treatment duration (months)**	**Primary outcome (FIT vs placebo)**	**Secondary outcome (FIT vs placebo)**
Lin et al. [115]	RCT	122	HTN (65%), DM (40%)	AVF	40 min FIT, 3 times weekly	Placebo	12	Rate of AVF malfunction within 12 months (thrombosis, intervention required) *12% vs 29%, $p = 0.02$*	Cumulative primary unassisted AVF patency *87% vs 70%, $p = 0.01$* Physiologic AVF maturation *82% vs 60% $p = 0.008$*
Lin et al. [116]	RCT	145	HTN (54%), DM (33%)	AVF	40 min FIT, 3 times weekly	Placebo	12	Effect of FIT on access flow at 12 months *13.2 ± 114.7 vs 33.4 ± 132.3 ml/min, $p < 0.021$* AVF malfunction *12.9% vs 30.1%, $p < 0.01$* AVF unassisted patency *85.9% vs 67.6%, $p < 0.01$*	NR

Perivascular application of recombinant elastase

Trial	Study	Number of participants	Co-morbidities	Access type	Intervention	Control	Treatment follow-up (months)	Primary outcome (PRT-201 vs placebo)	Secondary outcomes (PRT-201 vs placebo)
Dwivedi et al. [118]	RCT	89	DM (44%), HTN (40%)	AVG	Single dose escalation of low (0.01, 0.03 mg), medium (0.1, 0.3, 1.0 mg) and high (3.0, 6.0, 9.0 mg) PRT-201 immediately at AVG placement	Placebo	12	Safety (adverse events) 13% vs 14%, NS >/−25% increase in outflow vein diameter intraoperatively *33% vs 15%, high, $p = 0.052$*	Percentage change in intraoperative outflow vein diameter *Low 13%, $p = 0.01$; medium 15% $p = 0.070$; high 12%, $p < 0.001$; vs 5% placebo* Percentage change in intraoperative blood flow volume *Low 19%, $p = 0.34$; medium 36%, $p = 0.09$, high 46%, $p = 0.02$; vs 15% placebo*
Hye et al. [117]	RCT	151	CAD (55%), DM (45%), HTN (28%), PVD (24%), CVD (20%)	AVF	PRT-201 at 0.01 mg or 0.03 mg applied once to newly formed AVF	Placebo	12	Unassisted primary patency at 12 months *10 mcg vs placebo; HR 0.69, 95% CI 0.39–1.22, $p = 0.19$* *30 mcg vs placebo; HR 0.67, 95% CI 0.38–1.19, $p = 0.17$*	Secondary patency at 12 months *10 mcg vs placebo; HR 0.79, 95% CI 0.33–1.92, $p = 0.61$ 30 mcg vs placebo; HR 0.76, 95% CI 0.31–1.89, $p = 0.55$* Unassisted maturation at 3 months *10 mcg 67%, 30 mcg 70% vs placebo 54%, NS* Luminal stenosis (hemodynamically significant) at 3 months *10 mcg 41%, 30 mcg 35% vs placebo 40%, NS*

Vascugel

Trial	Study	Number of participants	Co-morbidities	Access type	Intervention	Control	Treatment follow-up (months)	Primary outcome (Vascugel vs placebo)	Secondary outcomes (Vascugel vs placebo)
Conte et al. [121]	Phase I/II clinical study	57	CAD (100%), DM (68%), Dyslipidemia (51%)	AVF (47%) AVG (53%)	Vascugel placement at newly formed access	Placebo	6	Safety at 30 days (incidence of infection, intervention and thrombosis) *10.9% vs 21.1%, NS*	Primary patency **AVG** *38% vs 23%, NS* **AVF** *60% vs 62%, NS* Assisted primary patency **AVG** *72% vs 58%, NS* **AVF** *96% vs 88%, NS*

Antiproliferative agents—COLL-R (drug-eluted combination product of collagen membrane and sirolimus)

Trial	Study	Number of participants	Co-morbidities	Access type	Intervention	Control	Treatment follow-up (months)	Primary outcome	Secondary outcomes
Paulson et al. [122]	Phase II clinical study	12	HTN (83%), DM (8%)	AVG	Surgical placement of PTFE grafts and COLL-R	NR	24	Safety (freedom from device related adverse events) *Endpoint met, nil adverse events*	Pharmacokinetics of sirolimus release *Whole blood sirolimus levels reached a mean peak of 4.8 ng/mL at 6 h and were less than 1 ng/mL at 1 week* Success of COLL-R implantation *100% success* Primary unassisted graft patency *75% at 12 months and 38% at 24 months*

DOI: http://dx.doi.org/10.5772/intechopen.83525

Trial	Study	Number of participants	Co-morbidities	Access type	Intervention	Control	Treatment follow-up (months)	Primary outcomes (PCB vs HPB)	Secondary outcomes (PCB vs HPB)
Paclitaxel-coated balloon angioplasty									
Kitrou et al. [123]	RCT	40	NR	AVF	PCB treatment of failing AVF	HPB	12	Device success *35% vs 100%, $p < 0.001$* Anatomic success *100% both groups* Clinical success *100% both groups* Target lesion revascularization-free survival *PCB 308 days; HPB 161 days; HR 0.478; 95% CI 0.236–0.966, $p = 0.03$*	Dialysis circuit primary patency *PCB 270 days; HPB 161 days; HR 0.479; 95% CI 0.237–0.968; $p = 0.04$* Procedure related complications *Nil*
Katsanos et al. [124]	RCT	40	DM (20%), HTN (13%)	AVF (35%), AVG (65%)	PCB treatment of failing access	HPB	6	Primary patency of treated lesion *70% vs 25% $p < 0.001$, HR 0.30, 95% CI 0.12–0.71, $p = 0.006$* Device success *45% vs 100%, $p < 0.001$* Procedural success *100% both groups*	Dialysis circuit survival *95% vs 90%, $p = 0.274$; HR 0.33, 95% CI 0.03 to 3.36, $p = 0.349$*

RCT, randomized controlled trial; HTN, hypertension; DM, diabetes mellitus; CAD, coronary artery disease; PVD, peripheral vascular disease; CHD, congestive heart disease; CVD, cerebrovascular disease; AVF, arteriovenous fistula; AVG arteriovenous graft; mg, milligrams; RR, relative risk; CI, confidence interval; NR, not reported; OR, odds ratio; HR, hazard ratio; IRR, incident rate ratio; SEM, standard error of the mean; NS, not significant; HD, hemodialysis; ACEI, angiotensin-converting enzyme inhibition; ARB, angiotensin II typ. 1 receptor blockers; pSLOT, piggybacking straight-line onlay technique; SLOT, side-to-side straight-line onlay technique; ETS, end-to-side; FIT, far infrared therapy; PRT-201, perivascular application of recombinant elastase; PTFE, polytetrafluoroethylene; PCB, paclitaxel-coated balloon angioplasty; HPB, high pressure balloon angioplasty.

Table 1.
Summary of trial results of systemic medical therapies and local interventions on vascular access outcomes in hemodialysis patients.

placebo (32% vs 72%, odds ratio [OR] 0.18, 95% confidence interval [CI] 0.05–0.66, $p < 0.01$) after a mean follow-up of 5 months [67]. In contrary, a randomized, double-blind, placebo-controlled parallel group study [69] assessing the effect of dipyridamole and/or aspirin on AVG thrombosis showed a non-significant increase in thrombosis in 10 of 20 patients (50%) treated with 325 mg of aspirin daily compared to 6 of 19 (32%) patients on placebo (relative risk [RR] 1.99, 95% CI 0.88–4.48, $p = 0.18$) over a 18-month follow-up period. Inconsistent outcomes have also been described for aspirin used for prevention of AVF failure. In a study of 92 participants [68] randomized to 1000 mg of aspirin on alternate days over a 28 day period or placebo, the frequency of AVF thrombosis was reduced more than 4-fold by aspirin compared to placebo (2 of 45 [4.4%] vs 11 of 47 [23.4%], $p < 0.05$). However, the most recent and largest RCT showed no significant reduction in AVF failure at 12 months in 488 patients randomized to receive 100 mg of aspirin or placebo for 3 months following AVF creation. AVF failure was defined as a composite of AVF thrombosis, AVF abandonment and cannulation failure [5]. Neither the composite binary outcome (45% participants treated with aspirin vs 43% treated with placebo, RR 1.05, 95% CI 0.84–1.31, $p = 0.68$) nor the individual outcome components were reduced by low-dose aspirin: AVF thrombosis (20% vs 18%, RR 1.09, 95% CI 0.72–1.64, $p = 0.70$), AVF abandonment (24% vs 18%, RR 1.31, 95% CI 0.89–1.95, $p = 0.17$) and cannulation failure (40% vs 39%, RR 0.99, 95% CI 0.76–1.27, $p = 0.92$) [5]. Differences in treatment dose, duration, sample size and outcome definition makes comparison of treatment efficacy across trials difficult. Considering the cumulative evidence to date, there remains considerable uncertainty as to whether aspirin reduces arteriovenous access failure.

4.1.1.2 Dipyridamole

Dipyridamole impairs platelet aggregation by inhibition of adenosine deaminase and phosphodiesterase, causing an increase of adenosine, adenine nucleotides and cyclic adenosine monophosphate (cAMP) levels [70]. As a phosphodiesterase inhibitor, it reduces vascular smooth muscle proliferation, and may prevent neointimal hyperplasia, stenosis and thrombosis of arteriovenous access [70, 71]. A randomized, double-blind, placebo-controlled parallel group study [69] of 107 patients with ESKD assessed the effect of dipyridamole (225 mg daily) and/or aspirin (325 mg daily) on the rate of AVG thrombosis over a treatment duration of 18 months (**Table 1**). The treatment groups were divided into two cohorts, type I which included patients with new AVGs (84 patients) vs type II which included patients with previously placed AVGs who had suffered graft thrombosis requiring thrombectomy or revision (23 patients). Dipyridamole reduced AVG thrombosis rates compared to placebo (RR 0.35, 95% CI 0.15–0.80, $p = 0.02$), used alone (17% vs 32%) or in combination with aspirin (23% vs 32%). A multicenter RCT involving 649 patients with new AVGs randomized individuals to dipyridamole (200 mg extended release twice daily) plus aspirin (25 mg twice daily) or placebo over 4.5 years with an additional 6-month follow-up [72]. At 12 months, the primary outcome of primary unassisted patency loss (patency without thrombosis or requirement of an intervention) occurred in 28% of patients treated with dipyridamole and aspirin compared to 23% receiving placebo (hazard ratio [HR] 0.82; 95% CI 0.68–0.98, $p = 0.03$) [72]. Pertaining to the evidence presented, dipyridamole alone or in combination with aspirin may be beneficial in preventing primary AVG failure.

4.1.1.3 Clopidogrel

Clopidogrel and ticlopidine are classed as thienopyridines. The active metabolite they produce irreversibly blocks the protein P2y12 component of the adenosine diphosphate (ADP) receptors on the platelet surface, preventing activation of the GPIIb/IIa receptor complex and reducing platelet aggregation [13]. The effects of clopidogrel (300 mg load followed by 75 mg daily) on access failure were evaluated in an RCT involving 877 patients undergoing AVF formation (**Table 1**). The rate of early fistula thrombosis (within 6 weeks) was lower with treatment (53 of 436 patients, 12.2%) compared to placebo (84 of the 430, 19.5%; RR 0.63, 95% CI 0.46–0.97, $p = 0.18$) [15], however, this benefit did not translate into an increase in the proportion of AVFs that became suitable for hemodialysis (61.8% vs 59.5%; RR 1.05, 95% CI 0.94–1.17, $p = 0.4$) [15]. A smaller RCT of 93 patients found that, compared with placebo, clopidogrel resulted in a lower risk of early fistula thrombosis (5.2% vs 21.6%; HR 0.72, 95% CI 0.41–1.01, $p = 0.03$) and a higher rate of first successful dialysis using the newly created AVF (92.3% vs 70.5%) [73]. In contrast, no benefit was identified from clopidogrel 75 mg and aspirin 325 mg vs placebo on graft thrombosis in an RCT involving 200 participants undergoing hemodialysis with newly formed AVGs (HR 0.81, 95% CI 0.47–1.40, $p = 0.45$) [74]. Considering the evidence to date, there remains uncertainty as to whether clopidogrel results in a clinically meaningful benefit beyond prevention of early thrombosis.

4.1.1.4 Ticlopidine

Three RCTs investigated the effects of ticlopidine on AVF thrombosis at 4 weeks (**Table 1**). Two small RCTs [75, 76] demonstrated that AVF thrombosis occurred in fewer patients receiving ticlopidine as compared with placebo. Grontoft et al. [75] studied 36 participants and showed that AVF thrombosis at 4 weeks was reduced in participants treated with 250 mg ticlopidine twice daily (11%) compared to placebo (47%, $p < 0.05$). In a pilot study of 18 participants [76], 250 mg ticlopidine given twice daily over 1 month resulted in half the thrombosis rates compared to placebo (25% vs 50% respectively). A multicenter RCT involving 250 participants [77] showed that ticlopidine did not significantly reduce AVF thrombosis compared to placebo at 4 weeks (12% vs 19%, OR 0.6, 95% CI 0.30–1.18, $p = 0.1$). A subsequent systematic review and meta-analysis of these trials [78] favored the use of ticlopidine in access thrombosis as a beneficial treatment (OR 0.45, 95% CI 0.25–0.82, $p = 0.009$).

A meta-analysis of 21 RCTs using any type of antiplatelet drug to prevent arteriovenous access failure demonstrated a 51% reduction in patency loss of AVFs with antiplatelet therapy compared to placebo (6 trials, 1222 participants, RR 0.49, 95% CI 0.30–0.81), while clinical benefits in preventing AVG thrombosis remained uncertain (3 trials, 956 participants, RR 0.94, 95% CI 0.80–1.10) [79].

Based on the available evidence, there may be a short-term benefit of antiplatelet agents in reducing arteriovenous access thrombosis [15, 78–80], though clinically meaningful benefits, including improved long-term patency or access usability for dialysis, have not been found [15, 79]. Therapeutic approaches targeting vascular remodeling and neointimal hyperplasia may be more beneficial in the longer term [13].

4.1.2 Omega-3 fatty acid supplementation (fish oil)

Omega-3 fatty acids (the active component of fish oil) are thought to reduce arteriovenous access thrombosis and improve maturation [81] through their antiproliferative [82], antiaggregatory [83], anti-inflammatory [84], antioxidant and vasodilatory effects [85–87].

Two RCTs have assessed the effect of fish oil on AVG patency (**Table 1**) [88, 89]. The largest study involved 196 patients with newly created AVGs treated with 4 g of fish oil or placebo for 12 months [89]. There was no statistically significant difference in the *proportion* of participants experiencing graft patency loss (thrombosis or radiological or surgical interventions) at 12 months between fish oil (48%) and placebo (62%, RR 0.78, 95% CI 0.60–1.03, p = 0.06). However, participants treated with fish oil experienced lower *rates* of loss of graft patency (incident rate ratio [IRR] 0.58, 95% CI 0.44–0.75), radiological or surgical interventions (IRR 0.59, 95% CI 0.44–0.78) and thrombotic events (IRR0.5, 95% CI 0.35–0.72). Another RCT including 24 patients randomized to treatment with fish oil or placebo for 12 months found that fish oil treatment led to greater primary patency (thrombosis free) after 12 months of follow-up (75.6% vs 14.9% respectively, p = 0.03) [88]. An RCT by Bowden et al. [90] was unable to replicate these findings in 29 participants, with no difference in the mean time to primary patency loss (thrombosis or venous outflow stenosis >50% requiring angioplasty) in the treatment group (254 ± 52 days, standard error of the mean [SEM] 51.8) compared to the placebo group (254 ± 35 days, SEM 34.6) over the 8-month follow-up period. The heterogeneity in outcome definitions (primary patency loss vs thrombosis) makes comparison across trials difficult. Although a risk reduction in graft thrombosis was described in a meta-analysis of data from four trials, this analysis incorporated events other than graft thrombosis including infection [86] and interventions [90]. When only including the trials that assessed the frequency of graft thrombosis [78], fish oil was no longer associated with a significant treatment benefit compared to placebo (OR 0.24; 95% CI, 0.03–1.95).

A large multicenter trial (Omega-3 fatty acids (fish oils) and aspirin in vascular access outcomes in renal disease [FAVORED]) [5] is the only RCT to date to examine the effect of fish oil on AVF failure. This trial included 567 patients with newly created AVF randomized to 4 g of fish oil daily or matching placebo for 3 months post AVF creation. At 12-month follow-up, no significant differences between the fish oil and placebo groups were identified for the primary composite outcome of AVF failure (47% identified in both groups, RR 1.03, 95% CI 0.86–1.23, p = 0.78) or for the individual components of the composite including AVF thrombosis (22% vs 23%, RR 0.98, 95% CI 0.72–1.34, p = 0.9), fistula abandonment (19% vs 22%, RR 0.87, 95% CI 0.62–1.2, p = 0.43) or cannulation failure (40% vs 39%, RR 1.03, 95% CI 0.83–1.26, p = 0.81) [5].

A recent meta-analysis of all RCTs (5 trials, 833 participants) evaluated the effect of fish oil supplementation in preventing arteriovenous access failure using standardized outcome definitions [81]. Key findings included that fish oil supplementation prevented primary patency loss with moderate certainty (RR 0.81, 95% CI 0.68–0.98), and that low quality evidence suggested that fish oil may have little effect on dialysis suitability failure (RR 0.95, 95% CI 0.73–1.23), access abandonment (RR 0.78, 95% CI 0.59–1.03), need for interventions (RR 0.82, 95% CI 0.64–1.04) or all-cause mortality (RR 0.99, 95% CI 0.51–1.92).

4.1.3 Statin therapy

Statins have been shown to reduce inflammation in the ESKD population, while also improving endothelial function beyond the effect of cholesterol lowering [91]. There is experimental evidence that statins reduce neointimal hyperplasia and vascular remodeling, which appears to be mediated by the reduction of vascular endothelial growth factor-A and matrix metalloproteinase (MMP) [92], and promotion of vasodilatation (via endothelial derived NO) [93].

An ancillary analysis of the Study of Heart and Renal Protection (SHARP) RCT comparing the effects of simvastatin/ezetimibe 20 mg/10 mg vs placebo on vascular access occlusive events (defined as any access revision procedure, access thrombosis, removal of an old dialysis access, or formation of new permanent dialysis access) in 2353 participants (94% AVF, 6% AVG) (**Table 1**) [94]. Simvastatin plus ezetimibe resulted in a 13% reduction in vascular occlusive events compared with placebo (RR 0.87, 95% CI 0.75–1.00, p = 0.05). Results were broadly similar for the individual components of the composite outcomes. However, the same group was unable to replicate this result in a post hoc analysis of the AURORA (A Study to Evaluate the Use of Rosuvastatin in Subjects on Regular Hemodialysis: An Assessment of Survival and Cardiovascular Events) trial cohort [94]. Specifically, occlusive vascular events were comparable between the rosuvastatin and placebo groups (28.9% vs 27.6%, respectively, RR 1.06, 95% CI 0.91–1.23, p = 0.44). When the SHARP and AURORA results were pooled, low density lipoprotein cholesterol (LDL-C) lowering therapy did not significantly reduce vascular occlusive events. These results were limited by the post hoc analysis of exploratory trial outcomes and the failure to include other large studies of cholesterol-lowering therapy (such as the Der Deutsche Diabetes Dialyze [4D] study [95]), such that results should be considered hypothesis-generating only.

Retrospective observational cohort analyses by Saran et al. [96] and Pisoni et al. [97] found statins were not beneficial in improving cumulative fistula survival. Specifically, statin therapy did not improve access maturation [97] or primary access patency [96]. Similarly, a retrospective review of 265 patients, of which 90% were on either simvastatin or atorvastatin, found that statin therapy did not affect the number of stenotic lesions in AVFs or time to primary angioplasty [91]. Whereas a case-control study of 60 dialysis patients receiving either folic acid and/or statin discovered improved primary patency in 35 patients with AVFs [34].

In summary, the evidence for benefits of statin use in the prevention of vascular access complications in hemodialysis patients is based on observational trial data and post hoc analysis of RCTs. To date, no RCT has been developed to determine the effect of statin therapy on primary patency rates in newly formed vascular access. There is currently insufficient evidence to support the routine use of statin therapy for preserving vascular access.

4.1.4 *Renin-angiotensin-aldosterone system blockers (angiotensin-converting enzyme inhibitors and angiotensin II type I receptor blockers)*

The renin-angiotensin-aldosterone system (RAAS) is an important modulator of the vascular smooth muscle cell proliferation that occurs in the intimal layer of the vein in response to injury [98]. Additionally, angiotensin II produced locally at the site of injury can induce growth factors that further promote vascular smooth muscle proliferation and a prothrombotic environment [98]. Blocking these pathways in animal models with the use of angiotensin-converting enzyme inhibition (ACEI) has been shown to prevent smooth muscle cell proliferation and migration [99, 100], inhibit intimal hyperplasia and extracellular matrix deposition [100–102], promote venous dilation [103] and prevent platelet activation [104, 105].

In the clinical setting, the effects of ACEI and/or angiotensin II type 1 receptor blockers (ARB) on primary and secondary arteriovenous access outcomes has been confined to retrospective observational cohort studies with conflicting findings (**Table 1**) [98, 99, 106–108]. A multi-center observational study by Sajgure et al. [98] compared the use of ACEI vs placebo on primary patency duration in AVGs (179 participants) and AVFs (87 participants) over a 24 month period. A longer primary patency duration was observed in the treatment AVG group compared with placebo (HR 0.48, 95% CI 0.31–0.73, p = 0.01), though no benefit was observed with the use of ACEI in AVFs (p = 0.45). Chen et al. [108] performed a retrospective analysis of the efficacy of ACEI and/or ARB therapy on primary patency loss of AVGs and AVFs in 42,244 patients over a 96-month period

(37,771 with AVFs [32.3% on an ACEI, 15% on an ARB], 4473 with AVGs [6.2% on an ACEI, 7.1% on an ARB]). ACEI use was associated with prolonged primary patency in both AVFs (HR 0.59, 95% CI 0.56–0.62, $p < 0.05$) and AVGs (HR 0.56, 95% CI 0.48–0.64, $p < 0.05$). Similarly, ARB use was shown to be beneficial in AVFs (HR 0.53, 95% CI 0.51–0.56, $p < 0.05$), and AVGs (HR0.54, 95% CI 0.47–0.61, $p < 0.05$) [108]. Furthermore, Jackson et al. [99] reported that ARB use prolonged 1- and 2-year primary patency in both, AVFs (55.2% at 1 year, 49.1% at 2 years; HR 0.35, 95% CI 0.16–0.76, $p = 0.008$) and AVGs (50.2% at 1 year, 29.7% at 2 years; HR0.41, 95% CI 0.18–0.95, $p = 0.039$). An international, prospective, observational study by Saran et al. [96] elucidated a clinically significant relationship between ACEI use and reduction in secondary AVF failure (RR 0.56, $p = 0.01$) and a trend toward improving primary AVF patency failure, while there was no significant treatment benefit in AVGs (primary RR 1.02, $p = 0.846$, secondary RR 1.16, $p = 0.133$). The same study found no significant benefit associated with the use of ARB in preventing primary or secondary patency failure in AVFs or AVGs. Available evidence is limited by substantial heterogeneity of treatment agents, dose, outcome definitions and study populations and unadjusted confounding associated with the observational study design. Randomized-controlled trials to confirm potential benefits of RAAS inhibitors are required.

4.1.5 Calcium channel blockers

Based on animal and human studies, calcium channel blockers (CCB) may inhibit neointimal hyperplasia [109, 110] and thereby reduce maturation failure [111] and restenosis post angioplasty [112]. In a prospective, observational study of 2313 participants (of which 970 were on CCB) [96], CCB use was associated with prolonged primary patency of AVGs (RR 0.86, $p = 0.034$), while no association with CCB was found for secondary AVG patency (RR 0.88, $p = 0.153$) as well as primary (RR 1.14, $p = 0.3$) and secondary AVF patency (RR 1.16, $p = 0.374$) (**Table 1**). A retrospective study by Chen et al. [108] including 42,244 patients (37,771 with AVFs [32.3% on a CCB], 4473 with AVGs [20.6% on a CCB]), described a significant relationship between CCB use and prolonged primary patency in both AVF (HR 0.485, CI 0.470–0.501) and AVG (HR 0.482, CI 0.442–0.526) groups. While there has currently been minimal investigation into the use of CCB in prevention of vascular access failure, further research may be warranted given the wide use of this antihypertensive agent in the hemodialysis population.

4.2 Local interventions

Targeted interventions to reduce upstream injury include new surgical techniques [113] and endovascular access creation [114], interventions to mitigate downstream responses include far infra-red therapy [115, 116], perivascular application of recombinant elastase [117, 118] and endothelial loaded gel foam wrap (Vascugel) [119–121], whereas antiproliferative agents including sirolimus [122] and paclitaxel [123, 124] have been developed to prevent neointimal hyperplasia and promote outward remodeling and vasodilatation [1, 13].

4.2.1 New surgical techniques to alter wall shear stress

Turbulent low-flow with low shear stress at the anastomosis leads to endothelial dysfunction, increased oxidative stress and an inflammatory and prothrombotic state, promoting AVF/AVG inward remodeling and neointimal hyperplasia [16, 125]. Optimization of flow dynamics through novel surgical techniques aimed at changing the anatomical configuration is a potential strategy to minimize this injury [17]. Baharat et al. [126] compared the use of the piggybacking Straight-Line Onlay Technique (pSLOT) to the traditional end-to-side (ETS) and side-to-side Straight-Line Onlay Techniques (SLOT), in a study of 125 patients (**Table 1**). They found a significant reduction in juxta-anastomotic stenosis using the novel pSLOT (3.7%) compared to traditional methods of ETS (14%) and SLOT (8.3%) ($p = 0.04$). This was accompanied by a significant reduction in overall fistula failure (pSLOT 16.7%, ETS 40.3%, SLOT 33.3%, $p = 0.01$) over the median 19-month follow-up.

The Optiflow Vascular Anastomotic device is a sutureless device that is able to provide reproducible anastomosis at a controlled geometry of 60° between the artery and vein, resulting in reduced surgical time, and optimized flow patterns and shear stress [13, 113], with a likely capability of shielding the perianastomotic region and preventing stenosis with its prosthetic material [13, 113]. This device is thought to clinically improve both vascular access maturation and patency [13]. Manson et al. [113] demonstrated safety and technical practicality in a human pilot study involving 10 patients. Subsequently, a prospective study of 41 patients performed at two centers by Chemla et al. [127] evaluated the maturation, patency, and safety of AVF using the Optiflow device. Unassisted maturation (defined as an outflow vein >/= 5 mm in diameter and flow >/= 500 ml/min not requiring intervention to maintain or promote maturation) was achieved in 72% of AVFs at 42 days and 68% at 90 days, unassisted patency in 88% of AVFs at 42 days and 78% at 90 days, and no serious device-related adverse events were reported [127]. In summary, the Optiflow device has shown promise in very small sample sizes and requires further evaluation in an RCT that is powered to confirm these clinical benefits.

4.2.2 Endovascular AVF creation

The creation of an AVF with an endovascular approach using a radiofrequency magnetic catheter-based system is suggested to cause less vessel trauma, resulting in a reduced stimulus for the formation of neointimal hyperplasia [13, 128]. Clinically this has the potential to translate into improved vascular access maturation and patency [13]. A prospective, single-arm, multicenter study (Novel Endovascular Access Trial [NEAT]) enrolled 80 patients (57% pre-dialysis and 43% on dialysis) who underwent endovascular arteriovenous anastomosis creation (**Table 1**) [114]. The AVF was successfully created in 98% of participants (95% CI 91–100%). Physiologically suitable AVF dialysis, defined as a brachial artery flow ≥500 mL/min and vein diameter ≥ 4 mm within 3 months, was achieved in 87% of participants (95% CI 75–94%) and 64% (95% CI 48–78%) were able to receive prescribed hemodialysis through the AVF using two-needle cannulation. Primary patency at 12 months was 69% (95% CI 54–79%) and cumulative patency 84% (95% CI 71–91%), and 24 secondary AVF interventions were required in 19 participants (0.46/patient-year). Serious procedure-related adverse events (access-site management, hemostasis and pseudoaneurysm) occurred in 8% of participants. These results suggest that endovascular AVF creation may be a viable, minimally invasive alternative for creating vascular access. However, long-term outcomes are currently lacking and comparison to open surgical techniques in a randomized controlled fashion may be difficult due to the unique location and type of vessels used for AVF.

4.2.3 Far infrared therapy

Infrared radiation is an invisible electromagnetic wave, with wavelengths ranging from 5.6 to 1000 μm [17]. This energy is perceived as heat by the thermoreceptors in the surrounding skin [116]. Far infrared therapy (FIT) has been shown to inhibit vascular smooth muscle cell proliferation and platelet aggregation [116], promote vasodilation [129], improve endothelial function [130] and reduce oxidative stress [13]. These pleiotropic effects upon vascular biology may be beneficial in improving maturation and vascular patency [13, 116]. An RCT by Lin et al. [116] involving 145 hemodialysis patients evaluated the effect of FIT on access blood flow and unassisted patency in native AVFs over a 12-month period (**Table 1**). Compared to placebo, FIT resulted in increased blood flow (13.2 ± 114.7 vs 33.4 ± 132.3 ml/min, $p < 0.021$) and unassisted patency (85.9% vs 67.6% respectively, $p < 0.01$) [116]. Additionally, Lin et al. [115] conducted an RCT involving 122 patients with advanced CKD pre-dialysis who underwent AVF creation. FIT applied for 40 min three times a week for 12 months, resulted in lower rates of AVF malfunction (thrombosis or requirement of intervention) compared with placebo (12% vs 29% respectively $p = 0.02$), higher maturation rates (82% vs 60% $p = 0.008$), and higher rates of cumulative unassisted AVF patency (87% vs 70% $p = 0.01$) at 12 months [115]. A subsequent meta-analysis of RCTs and quasi-RCTs by Wan et al. [131] included 21 studies and 1899 patients of whom 960 were treated with FIT. The result of this meta-analysis demonstrated that FIT improved primary AVF patency (pooled risk ratio [PRR] 1.24; 95% CI 1.12–1.37, $p < 0.001$), improved vascular access blood flow (mean difference [MD], 81.69 ml/min; 95% CI 46.17–117.21, $p < 0.001$), superior vascular access diameter level compared to control (MD 0.36 mm; 95% CI, 0.22–0.51, $p < 0.001$) and reduced AVF occlusion rates (PRR 0.2; 95% CI 0.08–0.46, $p < 0.001$) [131]. The quality of evidence provided in this meta-analysis is limited by small-scale studies of short duration (maximum 12 months). Given the convenience of FIT application during dialysis sessions and its non-invasive nature, this treatment strategy warrants further study to confirm the proposed benefits in improving vascular access maturation and patency.

4.2.4 Perivascular application of recombinant elastase

Elastin is a protein that provides blood vessels with their elasticity enabling control of vessel diameter [132]. Recombinant human type-1 pancreatic elastase (PRT-201) preferentially cleaves the peptide bonds abundant in elastin [133, 134]. Fragmentation of elastin leads to vasodilation and inhibits migration of adventitial myofibroblasts into the intimal layer [13, 135]. The rationale behind the use of PRT-201 is the theoretical assumption that application after AVF creation should destroy the elastin in the arteries and veins thereby resulting in faster AVF dilatation and maturation [1, 13]. Due to difficulties with inactivation of the enzyme following systemic administration, PRT-201 needs to be applied locally during surgery to provide targeted antiprotease effect [136]. Animal studies reported an increase in vessel diameter, blood flow, and inhibition of intimal hyperplasia with use of PRT-201 [137, 138]. An RCT [118] of 89 patients comparing low (0.01, 0.03 mg), medium (0.1, 0.3, 1.0 mg) and high (3.0, 6.0, 9.0 mg) dose PRT-201 vs placebo applied during AVG creation reported a larger percentage increase in outflow vein diameter intraoperatively with PRT-201 (5% placebo vs 13% [$p = 0.01$], 15% [$p = 0.070$], 12% [$p < 0.001$] in the low, medium and high dose groups, respectively) (**Table 1**). In contrast, only high dose PRT-201 led to a significant increase in blood flow compared to placebo (15% placebo vs 19% [$p = 0.34$], 36% [$p = 0.09$], 46% [$p = 0.02$], low, medium and high doses respectively) [118]. Conversely, a double-blind, randomized, placebo-controlled trial of a single local application of PRT-201 in 151 patients with advanced kidney disease undergoing AVF creation found no significant difference in unassisted primary patency over 1 year with low dose PRT compared to placebo (HR 0.69, 95% CI 0.39–1.22, $p = 0.19$ for 10 μg PRT-201 and HR 0.67, 95% CI 0.38–1.19, $p = 0.17$ for 30 μg PRT-201) [117]. While there is a potential immediate effect of high dose PRT-201 on intraoperative vein outflow diameter and blood flow, clinically meaningful long-term outcomes have not yet been addressed in adequately powered RCTs.

4.2.5 Endothelial loaded gel foam wrap (Vascugel)

Vascugel is an endothelial-cell-loaded wrap comprising a gel foam with allogeneic aortic endothelial cells [1, 53, 121]. Vascugel mediates its effects through the local delivery of "functional" endothelial cells at the anastomosis to promote outward vascular remodeling and prevent neointimal hyperplasia [1]. Preclinical studies involving porcine models of AVF and AVG have reported that local application of Vascugel resulted in a reduction in thrombus formation and vessel wall inflammation, an increase in luminal diameter and outward remodeling accompanied by reductions in MMP-2 expression, neovascularization and adventitial fibrosis [119, 120]. A phase II trial by Conte et al. [121] suggested that the use of Vascugel was a safe approach for local response to injury control at anastomotic sites, although it did not significantly affect primary and assisted patency rates in treated AVF and AVG compared with placebo (**Table 1**). A retrospective analysis of this trial showed an improved primary patency when Vascugel was used in AVGs of diabetic patients ($p = 0.05$), although the results of such a post hoc analysis should be interpreted with caution [53]. In summary, Vascugel has been identified as a safe intervention, though its clinical benefit on vascular access function has not been consistently demonstrated in human trials. Adequately powered RCTs investigating its clinical application are still needed.

4.2.6 Antiproliferative agents: COLL-R (drug-eluted combination product of collagen membrane and sirolimus)

Sirolimus (rapamycin) is an antiproliferative agent with immunosuppressive, anti-inflammatory and antiproliferative effects [139, 140], that has been shown to reduce vascular smooth muscle cell proliferation [13] and neointimal hyperplasia in vascular access [122]. When delivered locally, sirolimus reduces neointimal hyperplasia in coronary re-stenosis [1, 141–143]. COLL-R is a drug-eluted combination product of sirolimus and a collagen membrane, which can be implanted around the adventitial surface either at the arteriovenous anastomosis of the AVF or at the graft-vein anastomosis of the AVG [1, 13, 122]. Sirolimus is then eluted from the COLL-R, inhibiting neointimal proliferation at the anastomosis [122], translating clinically to a potential improvement in vascular access maturation and patency [13]. A single-arm phase II study by Paulson et al. [122] containing a cohort of 12 hemodialysis patients undergoing AVG formation with intraoperative COLL-R placement demonstrated primary unassisted patency rates of 75% at 12 months and 38% at 24 months and a thrombosis rate of 0.37 episodes per patient year (**Table 1**) [122]. In a sub-group of 5 patients, whole blood sirolimus levels reached a mean peak of 4.8 ng/mL at 6 h and were less than 1 ng/mL at 1 week. Results from a phase III RCT evaluating AVF suitability for dialysis at 6 months with and without a perivascular Sirolimus-Eluting Collagen Implant are currently awaited (NCT02513303).

4.2.7 Paclitaxel-coated balloon angioplasty

Drug-eluting balloons can deliver antiproliferative agents (such as paclitaxel) at angioplasty sites and thereby reduce neointimal hyperplasia and restenosis following endothelial injury caused by the angioplasty [1, 144]. Paclitaxel-coated balloon (PCB) angioplasty has been successfully used to treat coronary stenosis [145] and peripheral vascular disease [146]. In 40 patients with stenotic AVFs and AVGs, PCB angioplasty resulted in better target lesion and circuit primary patency rates at 6 months compared to high pressure balloon (HPB) angioplasty (70% vs 25% respectively, $p < 0.001$) [124] . Lai et al. [147] also reported improved AVF patency rate at 6 months in 10 patients (70% vs 0%, $p < 0.01$) although this was no longer statistically significant at 12 months (20% vs 0%, $P > 0.05$). A subsequent single center RCT by Kitou et al. [123] randomized 40 patients to receive PCB angioplasty or HPB angioplasty for dysfunctional AVFs, with a 12-month follow-up (**Table 1**). Primary endpoints included device success, anatomic success, clinical success and target lesion revascularization-free survival with secondary endpoints of dialysis circuit primary patency and procedure related complications [123]. Use of PCB angioplasty in dysfunctional AVFs resulted in superior target lesion revascularization-free survival (PCB 308 days; HPB 161 days; HR 0.478; 95% CI 0.236–0.966, $p = 0.03$) and dialysis access circuit primary patency (PCB 270 days; HPB 161 days; HR 0.479; 95% CI 0.237–0.968; $p = 0.04$) in comparison to HPB angioplasty, though, additional HPB post dilatation was required in 65% of cases. Current trial results support the use of PCB angioplasty to prevent re-stenosis in AVF. However, higher costs compared to conventional angioplasty and the lack of larger RCTs currently prevent its routine use in clinical practice.

5. Process of care and individualization

Systemic and local therapies to improve arteriovenous access outcomes have been limited, as outlined above. A multipronged approach including optimization of process of care may be more powerful to increase the use of AVFs or AVGs, as opposed to CVCs, than a single therapeutic intervention. An integrated approach to arteriovenous access care which included nephrologists, vascular surgeons, radiologists, access coordinators, and scheduled access procedures with tracked outcomes was demonstrated by Allon et al. [148] to reduce complications associated with surgical access procedures. These benefits included a 60% decreased rate of AVG thrombosis, improved graft secondary patency procedures, and an increase in the AVF creation rate from 33 to 69%. Arora et al. [149] found that patients who were referred to a nephrologist at least 4 months prior to dialysis initiation were 10 times more likely to have a successful functioning access at the first dialysis session, with 40% in the early referral group initiating dialysis with permanent vascular access (80% AVFs, 20% AVGs) vs 4% in the late referral group. This was supported by Roubicek at el [150] who found that 53% of patients referred early for arteriovenous access creation had functional AVFs vs 12% who were referred late. Having a vascular access coordinator can improve the number of AVFs created and decrease vascular access-related hospitalizations and infections [151]. Other strategies, including vein preservation policies, patient education regarding vein protection and access care, preoperative vein mapping and timely access creation have been found to increase fistula prevalence, decrease primary vascular access failure and increase cumulative patency [152–154]. The literature suggest that superior arteriovenous access success is achieved when the AVF is created by a skilled vascular surgeon, [45–49], with the emphasis being placed on the number of AVFs created over the total years of training [48, 50]. In the post-operative setting, timely assessment of arteriovenous access at 4 weeks is recommended to ensure access function is adequate, and to enable early surgical or endovascular intervention to prevent or treat primary access failure. Finally, arteriovenous access cannulation by appropriately trained staff has been shown to prolong AVF survival, while also minimizing the risk of infection.

6. Conclusion and future direction

The medical community's understanding of the pathology and pathogenesis of vascular access dysfunction has improved dramatically in recent times and enabled the development of novel targeted treatment approaches. The combination of interventions focusing on upstream events (i.e. optimization of hemodynamics and reduction in vascular injury through surgical/endovascular techniques) and downstream pathways (antiproliferative and anti-inflammatory therapies) may be a promising treatment approach to be assessed in future trials. Emphasis of a multipronged approach including optimization of process of care, education, surgical skills and surveillance combined with targeted therapies may yield the best outcomes and should be evaluated with innovative trial designs.

Conflict of interest

The authors have no conflict of interest to declare.

Author details

Rebecca Hudson[1], David Johnson[1,2,3*] and Andrea Viecelli[1,2]

1 Department of Nephrology, Princess Alexandra Hospital, Brisbane, Australia

2 Centre for Kidney Disease Research, University of Queensland, Brisbane, Australia

3 Translational Research Institute, Brisbane, Australia

*Address all correspondence to: david.johnson2@health.qld.gov.au

References

[1] Riella MC, Roy-Chaudhury P. Vascular access in haemodialysis: Strengthening the Achilles' heel. Nature Reviews. Nephrology. 2013;**9**(6): 348-357

[2] Broumand B. Diabetes: Changing the fate of diabetics in the dialysis unit. Blood Purification. 2007;**25**(1):39-47

[3] Levin A, Tonelli M, Bonventre J, Coresh J, Donner JA, Fogo AB, et al. Global kidney health 2017 and beyond: A roadmap for closing gaps in care, research, and policy. Lancet. 2017; **390**(10105):1888-1917

[4] Bello AK, Levin A, Tonelli M, Okpechi IG, Feehally J, Harris D, et al. Assessment of global kidney health care status. Journal of the American Medical Association. 2017;**317**(18): 1864-1881

[5] Irish AB, Viecelli AK, Hawley CM, Hooi LS, Pascoe EM, Paul-Brent PA, et al. Effect of fish oil supplementation and aspirin use on Arteriovenous fistula failure in patients requiring hemodialysis: A randomized clinical trial. JAMA Internal Medicine. 2017; **177**(2):184-193

[6] Liyanage T, Ninomiya T, Jha V, Neal B, Patrice HM, Okpechi I, et al. Worldwide access to treatment for end-stage kidney disease: A systematic review. Lancet. 2015;**385**(9981): 1975-1982

[7] Beathard GA, Lok CE, Glickman MH, Al-Jaishi AA, Bednarski D, Cull DL, et al. Definitions and end points for interventional studies for arteriovenous dialysis access. Clinical Journal of the American Society of Nephrology. 2018; **13**(3):501-512

[8] Hemodialysis Adequacy Work G. Clinical practice guidelines for hemodialysis adequacy, update 2006. American Journal of Kidney Diseases. 2006;**48**(Supp. 1):S2-S90

[9] Viecelli AK, Pascoe E, Polkinghorne KR, Hawley C, Paul-Brent PA, Badve SV, et al. The Omega-3 fatty acids (fish oils) and aspirin in vascular access outcomes in renal disease (FAVOURED) study: The updated final trial protocol and rationale of post-initiation trial modifications. BMC Nephrology. 2015;**16**:89

[10] Polkinghorne KR, McDonald SP, Atkins RC, Kerr PG. Vascular access and all-cause mortality: A propensity score analysis. Journal of the American Society of Nephrology. 2004;**15**(2): 477-486

[11] Allon M, Robbin ML. Increasing arteriovenous fistulas in hemodialysis patients: Problems and solutions. Kidney International. 2002;**62**(4): 1109-1124

[12] Lok CE, Sontrop JM, Tomlinson G, Rajan D, Cattral M, Oreopoulos G, et al. Cumulative patency of contemporary fistulas versus grafts (2000–2010). Clinical Journal of the American Society of Nephrology. 2013;**8**(5):810-818

[13] Viecelli AK, Mori TA, Roy-Chaudhury P, Polkinghorne KR, Hawley CM, Johnson DW, et al. The pathogenesis of hemodialysis vascular access failure and systemic therapies for its prevention: Optimism unfulfilled. Seminars in Dialysis. 2018;**31**(3):244-257

[14] Miller PE, Carlton D, Deierhoi MH, Redden DT, Allon M. Natural history of arteriovenous grafts in hemodialysis patients. American Journal of Kidney Diseases. 2000;**36**(1):68-74

[15] Dember LM, Beck GJ, Allon M, Delmez JA, Dixon BS, Greenberg A,

et al. Effect of clopidogrel on early failure of arteriovenous fistulas for hemodialysis: A randomized controlled trial. Journal of the American Medical Association. 2008;**299**(18):2164-2171

[16] Roy-Chaudhury P, Sukhatme VP, Cheung AK. Hemodialysis vascular access dysfunction: A cellular and molecular viewpoint. Journal of the American Society of Nephrology. 2006; **17**(4):1112-1127

[17] Roy-Chaudhury P, Kruskat L. Future direction for vascular access for hemodialysis. Seminars in Dialysis. 2014;**28**(2):107-113

[18] Manns B, Tonelli M, Yilmaz S, Lee H, Laupland K, Klarenbach S, et al. Establishment and maintenance of vascular access in incident hemodialysis patients: A prospective cost analysis. Journal of the American Society of Nephrology. 2005;**16**(1):201-209

[19] Feldman HI, Kobrin S, Wasserstein A. Hemodialysis vascular access morbidity. Journal of the American Society of Nephrology. 1996;**7**(4): 523-535

[20] Feldman HI, Held PJ, Hutchinson JT, Stoiber E, Hartigan MF, Berlin JA. Hemodialysis vascular access morbidity in the United States. Kidney International. 1993;**43**(5):1091-1096

[21] Tong A, Manns B, Hemmelgarn B, Wheeler DC, Evangelidis N, Tugwell P, et al. Establishing core outcome domains in hemodialysis: Report of the Standardized Outcomes in Nephrology-Hemodialysis (SONG-HD) Consensus Workshop. American Journal of Kidney Diseases. 2017;**69**(1):97-107

[22] Lu DY, Chen EY, Wong DJ, Yamamoto K, Protack CD, Williams WT, et al. Vein graft adaptation and fistula maturation in the arterial environment. The Journal of Surgical Research. 2014;**188**(1):162-173

[23] Arer IM, Yabanoglu H. Impact of surgeon factor on radiocephalic fistula patency rates. Annals of Medicine and Surgery (Lond). 2016;**5**:86-89

[24] Puskar D, Pasini J, Savic I, Bedalov G, Sonicki Z. Survival of primary arteriovenous fistula in 463 patients on chronic hemodialysis. Croatian Medical Journal. 2002;**43**(3):306-311

[25] Miller CD, Robbin ML, Allon M. Gender differences in outcomes of arteriovenous fistulas in hemodialysis patients. Kidney International. 2003; **63**(1):346-352

[26] Jennings WC, Landis L, Taubman KE, Parker DE. Creating functional autogenous vascular access in older patients. Journal of Vascular Surgery. 2011;**53**(3):713-719; discussion 9

[27] Diehm N, van den Berg JC, Schnyder V, Buhler J, Willenberg T, Widmer M, et al. Determinants of haemodialysis access survival. VASA Journal. 2010;**39**(2):133-139

[28] Marcus RJ, Marcus DA, Sureshkumar KK, Hussain SM, McGill RL. Gender differences in vascular access in hemodialysis patients in the United States: Developing strategies for improving access outcome. Gender Medicine. 2007;**4**(3):193-204

[29] Caplin N, Sedlacek M, Teodorescu V, Falk A, Uribarri J. Venous access: Women are equal. American Journal of Kidney Diseases. 2003;**41**(2):429-432

[30] Chitalia N, Ross L, Krishnamoorthy M, Kapustin A, Shanahan CM, Kaski JC, et al. Neointimal hyperplasia and calcification in medium sized arteries in adult patients with chronic kidney disease. Seminars in Dialysis. 2015; **28**(3):E35-E40

[31] Woods JD, Turenne MN, Strawderman RL, Young EW, Hirth RA, Port FK, et al. Vascular access survival among incident hemodialysis patients in the United States. American Journal of Kidney Diseases. 1997;**30**(1):50-57

[32] Zarins CK, Zatina MA, Giddens DP, Ku DN, Glagov S. Shear stress regulation of artery lumen diameter in experimental atherogenesis. Journal of Vascular Surgery. 1987;**5**(3):413-420

[33] Dixon BS. Why don't fistulas mature? Kidney International. 2006; **70**(8):1413-1422

[34] Righetti M, Ferrario G, Serbelloni P, Milani S, Tommasi A. Some old drugs improve late primary patency rate of native arteriovenous fistulas in hemodialysis patients. Annals of Vascular Surgery. 2009;**23**(4):491-497

[35] Kim YO, Song HC, Yoon SA, Yang CW, Kim NI, Choi YJ, et al. Preexisting intimal hyperplasia of radial artery is associated with early failure of radiocephalic arteriovenous fistula in hemodialysis patients. American Journal of Kidney Diseases. 2003;**41**(2):422-428

[36] Beks PJ, Mackaay AJ, de Neeling JN, de Vries H, Bouter LM, Heine RJ. Peripheral arterial disease in relation to glycaemic level in an elderly Caucasian population: The Hoorn study. Diabetologia. 1995;**38**(1):86-96

[37] Konner K. Primary vascular access in diabetic patients: An audit. Nephrology, Dialysis, Transplantation. 2000;**15**(9):1317-1325

[38] Ravani P, Marcelli D, Malberti F. Vascular access surgery managed by renal physicians: The choice of native arteriovenous fistulas for hemodialysis. American Journal of Kidney Diseases. 2002;**40**(6):1264-1276

[39] Peterson WJ, Barker J, Allon M. Disparities in fistula maturation persist despite preoperative vascular mapping. Clinical Journal of the American Society of Nephrology. 2008;**3**(2):437-441

[40] Miller PE, Tolwani A, Luscy CP, Deierhoi MH, Bailey R, Redden DT, et al. Predictors of adequacy of arteriovenous fistulas in hemodialysis patients. Kidney International. 1999; **56**(1):275-280

[41] Lok CE, Allon M, Moist L, Oliver MJ, Shah H, Zimmerman D. Risk equation determining unsuccessful cannulation events and failure to maturation in arteriovenous fistulas (REDUCE FTM I). Journal of the American Society of Nephrology. 2006; **17**(11):3204-3212

[42] Obialo CI, Tagoe AT, Martin PC, Asche-Crowe PE. Adequacy and survival of autogenous arteriovenous fistula in African American hemodialysis patients. ASAIO Journal. 2003;**49**(4):435-439

[43] Wilmink T, Wijewardane A, Lee K, Murley A, Hollingworth L, Powers S, et al. Effect of ethnicity and socioeconomic status on vascular access provision and performance in an urban NHS hospital. Clinical Kidney Journal. 2017;**10**(1):62-67

[44] Woo K, Gascue L, Goldman DP, Romley JA. Variations in outcomes of hemodialysis vascular access by race/ ethnicity in the elderly. Journal of Vascular Surgery. 2017;**65**(3):783-792 e4

[45] O'Hare AM, Dudley RA, Hynes DM, McCulloch CE, Navarro D, Colin P, et al. Impact of surgeon and surgical center characteristics on choice of permanent vascular access. Kidney International. 2003;**64**(2):681-689

[46] Huijbregts HJ, Bots ML, Moll FL, Blankestijn PJ, CIMINO members. Hospital specific aspects predominantly determine primary failure of hemodialysis arteriovenous fistulas.

Journal of Vascular Surgery. 2007;**45**(5):962-967

[47] He C, Charoenkul V, Kahn T, Langhoff E, Uribarri J, Sedlacek M. Impact of the surgeon on the prevalence of arteriovenous fistulas. ASAIO Journal. 2002;**48**(1):39-40

[48] Goodkin DA, Pisoni RL, Locatelli F, Port FK, Saran R. Hemodialysis vascular access training and practices are key to improved access outcomes. American Journal of Kidney Diseases. 2010;**56**(6):1032-1042

[49] Choi KL, Salman L, Krishnamurthy G, Mercado C, Merrill D, Thomas I, et al. Impact of surgeon selection on access placement and survival following preoperative mapping in the "Fistula First" era. Seminars in Dialysis. 2008;**21**(4):341-345

[50] Saran R, Elder SJ, Goodkin DA, Akiba T, Ethier J, Rayner HC, et al. Enhanced training in vascular access creation predicts arteriovenous fistula placement and patency in hemodialysis patients: Results from the Dialysis Outcomes and Practice Patterns Study. Annals of Surgery. 2008;**247**(5):885-891

[51] Kats M, Hawxby AM, Barker J, Allon M. Impact of obesity on arteriovenous fistula outcomes in dialysis patients. Kidney International. 2007;**71**(1):39-43

[52] Plumb TJ, Adelson AB, Groggel GC, Johanning JM, Lynch TG, Lund B. Obesity and hemodialysis vascular access failure. American Journal of Kidney Diseases. 2007;**50**(3):450-454

[53] Conte MS, Nugent HM, Gaccione P, Roy-Chaudhury P, Lawson JH. Influence of diabetes and perivascular allogeneic endothelial cell implants on arteriovenous fistula remodeling. Journal of Vascular Surgery. 2011;**54**(5):1383-1389

[54] Parisotto MT, Schoder VU, Miriunis C, Grassmann AH, Scatizzi LP, Kaufmann P, et al. Cannulation technique influences arteriovenous fistula and graft survival. Kidney International. 2014;**86**(4):790-797

[55] Tordoir J, Canaud B, Haage P, Konner K, Basci A, Fouque D, et al. EBPG on vascular access. Nephrology Dialysis Transplantation. 2007;**22**(Suppl_2):ii88-ii117

[56] Jindal K, Chan CT, Deziel C, Hirsch D, Soroka SD, Tonelli M, et al. Vascular access. Journal of the American Society of Nephrology. 2006;**17**(3 supp. 1):S16-S23

[57] Jindal K, Chan CT, Deziel C, Hirsch D, Soroka SD, Tonelli M, et al. Hemodialysis clinical practice guidelines for the Canadian Society of Nephrology. Journal of the American Society of Nephrology. 2006;**17**(3 supp. 1):S1

[58] Polkinghorne KR, Chin GK, MacGinley RJ, Owen AR, Russell C, Talaulikar GS, et al. KHA-CARI guideline: Vascular access—Central venous catheters, arteriovenous fistulae and arteriovenous grafts. Nephrology. 2013;**18**(11):701-705

[59] McCann M, Einarsdottir H, Van Waeleghem JP, Murphy F, Sedgwick J. Vascular access management II: AVF/AVG cannulation techniques and complications. Journal of Renal Care. 2009;**35**(2):90-98

[60] Feinfeld DA, Batista R, Mir R, Babich D. Changes in venous histology in chronic hemodialysis patients. American Journal of Kidney Diseases. 1999;**34**(4):702-705

[61] Falk A, Teodorescu V, Lou WY, Uribarri J, Vassalotti JA. Treatment of "swing point stenoses" in hemodialysis arteriovenous fistulae. Clinical Nephrology. 2003;**60**(1):35-41

[62] Shenoy S, Woodward RS. Economic impact of the beneficial effect of changing vascular anastomotic technique in hemodialysis access. Vascular and Endovascular Surgery. 2005;**39**(5):437-443

[63] Rothuizen TC, Wong C, Quax PH, van Zonneveld AJ, Rabelink TJ, Rotmans JI. Arteriovenous access failure: More than just intimal hyperplasia? Nephrology, Dialysis, Transplantation. 2013;**28**(5):1085-1092

[64] Cooke JP, Rossitch E Jr, Andon NA, Loscalzo J, Dzau VJ. Flow activates an endothelial potassium channel to release an endogenous nitrovasodilator. The Journal of Clinical Investigation. 1991; **88**(5):1663-1671

[65] Ene-Iordache B, Mosconi L, Antiga L, Bruno S, Anghileri A, Remuzzi G, et al. Radial artery remodeling in response to shear stress increase within arteriovenous fistula for hemodialysis access. Endothelium. 2003;**10**(2):95-102

[66] Langer S, Heiss C, Paulus N, Bektas N, Mommertz G, Rowinska Z, et al. Functional and structural response of arterialized femoral veins in a rodent AV fistula model. Nephrology, Dialysis, Transplantation. 2009;**24**(7):2201-2206

[67] Harter HR, Burch JW, Majerus PW, Stanford N, Delmez JA, Anderson CB, et al. Prevention of thrombosis in patients on hemodialysis by low-dose aspirin. The New England Journal of Medicine. 1979;**301**(11):577-579

[68] Andrassy K, Malluche H, Bornefeld H, Comberg M, Ritz E, Jesdinsky H, et al. Prevention of p.o. clotting of av. cimino fistulae with acetylsalicyl acid. Results of a prospective double blind study. Klinische Wochenschrift. 1974; **52**(7):348-349

[69] Sreedhara R, Himmelfarb J, Lazarus JM, Hakim RM. Anti-platelet therapy in graft thrombosis: Results of a prospective, randomized, double-blind study. Kidney International. 1994;**45**(5): 1477-1483

[70] Harker LA, Kadatz RA. Mechanism of action of dipyridamole. Thrombosis Research. Supplement. 1983;**4**:39-46

[71] Himmelfarb J, Couper L. Dipyridamole inhibits PDGF- and bFGF-induced vascular smooth muscle cell proliferation. Kidney International. 1997;**52**(6):1671-1677

[72] Dixon BS, Beck GJ, Vazquez MA, Greenberg A, Delmez JA, Allon M, et al. Effect of dipyridamole plus aspirin on hemodialysis graft patency. The New England Journal of Medicine. 2009; **360**(21):2191-2201

[73] Ghorbani A, Aalamshah M, Shahbazian H, Ehsanpour A, Aref A. Randomized controlled trial of clopidogrel to prevent primary arteriovenous fistula failure in hemodialysis patients. Indian Journal of Nephrology. 2009;**19**(2):57-61

[74] Kaufman JS, O'Connor TZ, Zhang JH, Cronin RE, Fiore LD, Ganz MB, et al. Randomized controlled trial of clopidogrel plus aspirin to prevent hemodialysis access graft thrombosis. Journal of the American Society of Nephrology. 2003;**14**(9):2313-2321

[75] Grontoft KC, Mulec H, Gutierrez A, Olander R. Thromboprophylactic effect of ticlopidine in arteriovenous fistulas for haemodialysis. Scandinavian Journal of Urology and Nephrology. 1985;**19**(1): 55-57

[76] Fiskerstrand CE, Thompson IW, Burnet ME, Williams P, Anderton JL. Double-blind randomized trial of the effect of ticlopidine in arteriovenous fistulas for hemodialysis. Artificial Organs. 1985;**9**(1):61-63

[77] Grontoft KC, Larsson R, Mulec H, Weiss LG, Dickinson JP. Effects of

ticlopidine in AV-fistula surgery in uremia. Fistula Study Group. Scandinavian Journal of Urology and Nephrology. 1998;**32**(4):276-283

[78] Tanner NC, Da Silva A. Medical adjuvant treatment to increase patency of arteriovenous fistulae and grafts. Cochrane Database of Systematic Reviews. 2015;7:CD002786

[79] Palmer SC, Di Micco L, Razavian M, Craig JC, Ravani P, Perkovic V, et al. Antiplatelet therapy to prevent hemodialysis vascular access failure: Systematic review and meta-analysis. American Journal of Kidney Diseases. 2013;**61**(1):112-122

[80] Kaufman JS. Antithrombotic agents and the prevention of access thrombosis. Seminars in Dialysis. 2000; **13**(1):40-46

[81] Viecelli AK, Irish AB, Polkinghorne KR, Hawley CM, Johnson DW, Mori TA, et al. Omega-3 polyunsaturated fatty acid supplementation to prevent arteriovenous fistula and graft failure: A systematic review and meta-analysis of randomized controlled trials. American Journal of Kidney Diseases. 2018;**72**(1): 50-61

[82] Fox PL, DiCorleto PE. Fish oils inhibit endothelial cell production of platelet-derived growth factor-like protein. Science. 1988;**241**(4864): 453-456

[83] Rylance PB, Gordge MP, Saynor R, Parsons V, Weston MJ. Fish oil modifies lipids and reduces platelet aggregability in haemodialysis patients. Nephron. 1986;**43**(3):196-202

[84] Calder PC. Omega-3 polyunsaturated fatty acids and inflammatory processes: Nutrition or pharmacology? British Journal of Clinical Pharmacology. 2013;**75**(3): 645-662

[85] Wang Q, Liang X, Wang L, Lu X, Huang J, Cao J, et al. Effect of omega-3 fatty acids supplementation on endothelial function: A meta-analysis of randomized controlled trials. Atherosclerosis. 2012;**221**(2):536-543

[86] Hung AM, Booker C, Ellis CD, Siew ED, Graves AJ, Shintani A, et al. Omega-3 fatty acids inhibit the up-regulation of endothelial chemokines in maintenance hemodialysis patients. Nephrology, Dialysis, Transplantation. 2015;**30**(2): 266-274

[87] Friedman A, Moe S. Review of the effects of omega-3 supplementation in dialysis patients. Clinical Journal of the American Society of Nephrology. 2006; **1**(2):182-192

[88] Schmitz PG, McCloud LK, Reikes ST, Leonard CL, Gellens ME. Prophylaxis of hemodialysis graft thrombosis with fish oil: Double-blind, randomized, prospective trial. Journal of the American Society of Nephrology. 2002;**13**(1):184-190

[89] Lok CE, Moist L, Hemmelgarn BR, Tonelli M, Vazquez MA, Dorval M, et al. Effect of fish oil supplementation on graft patency and cardiovascular events among patients with new synthetic arteriovenous hemodialysis grafts: A randomized controlled trial. Journal of the American Medical Association. 2012;**307**(17):1809-1816

[90] Bowden RG, Wilson RL, Gentile M, Ounpraseuth S, Moore P, Leutholtz BC. Effects of omega-3 fatty acid supplementation on vascular access thrombosis in polytetrafluorethylene grafts. Journal of Renal Nutrition. 2007; **17**(2):126-131

[91] Birch N, Fillaus J, Florescu MC. The effect of statin therapy on the formation of arteriovenous fistula stenoses and the rate of reoccurrence of previously treated stenoses. Hemodialysis International. 2013;**17**(4):586-593

[92] Janardhanan R, Yang B, Vohra P, Roy B, Withers S, Bhattacharya S, et al. Simvastatin reduces venous stenosis formation in a murine hemodialysis vascular access model. Kidney International. 2013;**84**(2):338-352

[93] Tsiara S, Elisaf M, Mikhailidis DP. Early vascular benefits of statin therapy. Current Medical Research and Opinion. 2003;**19**(6):540-556

[94] Herrington W, Emberson J, Staplin N, Blackwell L, Fellstrom B, Walker R, et al. The effect of lowering LDL cholesterol on vascular access patency: Post hoc analysis of the study of heart and renal protection. Clinical Journal of the American Society of Nephrology. 2014;**9**(5):914-919

[95] Wanner C, Krane V, Marz W, Olschewski M, Asmus HG, Kramer W, et al. Randomized controlled trial on the efficacy and safety of atorvastatin in patients with typ. 2 diabetes on hemodialysis (4D study): Demographic and baseline characteristics. Kidney & Blood Pressure Research. 2004;**27**(4): 259-266

[96] Saran R, Dykstra DM, Wolfe RA, Gillespie B, Held PJ, Young EW. Association between vascular access failure and the use of specific drugs: The Dialysis outcomes and practice patterns study (DOPPS). American Journal of Kidney Diseases. 2002;**40**(6):1255-1263

[97] Pisoni R, Barker-Finkel J, Allon M. Statin therapy is not associated with improved vascular access outcomes. Clinical Journal of the American Society of Nephrology. 2010;**5**(8):1447-1450

[98] Sajgure A, Choudhury A, Ahmed Z, Choudhury D. Angiotensin converting enzyme inhibitors maintain polytetrafluoroethylene graft patency. Nephrology, Dialysis, Transplantation. 2007;**22**(5):1390-1398

[99] Jackson RS, Sidawy AN, Amdur RL, Khetarpal A, Macsata RA. Angiotensin receptor blockers and antiplatelet agents are associated with improved primary patency after arteriovenous hemodialysis access placement. Journal of Vascular Surgery. 2011;**54**(6): 1706-1712

[100] Yamada T, Kondo T, Numaguchi Y, Tsuzuki M, Matsubara T, Manabe I, et al. Angiotensin II receptor blocker inhibits neointimal hyperplasia through regulation of smooth muscle-like progenitor cells. Arteriosclerosis, Thrombosis, and Vascular Biology. 2007;**27**(11):2363-2369

[101] O'Donohoe MK, Schwartz LB, Radic ZS, Mikat EM, McCann RL, Hagen PO. Chronic ACE inhibition reduces intimal hyperplasia in experimental vein grafts. Annals of Surgery. 1991;**214**(6):727-732

[102] Yagi S, Morita T, Katayama S. Combined treatment with an AT1 receptor blocker and angiotensin converting enzyme inhibitor has an additive effect on inhibiting neointima formation via improvement of nitric oxide production and suppression of oxidative stress. Hypertension Research. 2004;**27**(2):129-135

[103] Baan J Jr, Chang PC, Vermeij P, Pfaffendorf M, van Zwieten PA. Venoconstriction by angiotensin II in the human forearm is inhibited by losartan but not by nicardipine. Journal of Cardiovascular Pharmacology. 1998; **31**(1):50-55

[104] Kalinowski L, Matys T, Chabielska E, Buczko W, Malinski T. Angiotensin II AT1 receptor antagonists inhibit platelet adhesion and aggregation by nitric oxide release. Hypertension. 2002;**40**(4): 521-527

[105] Katoh M, Egashira K, Mitsui T, Chishima S, Takeshita A, Narita H. Angiotensin-converting enzyme inhibitor prevents plasminogen activator inhibitor-1 expression in a rat model with cardiovascular remodeling

induced by chronic inhibition of nitric oxide synthesis. Journal of Molecular and Cellular Cardiology. 2000;**32**(1): 73-83

[106] Moon JY, Jeong KH, Paik SS, Han JJ, Lee SH, Lee TW, et al. Arteriovenous fistula patency associated with angiotensin-converting enzyme I/D polymorphism and ACE inhibition or AT1 receptor blockade. Nephron. Clinical Practice. 2009;**111**(2): c110-c116

[107] Diskin CJ, Stokes TJ, Thomas SG, Ravis W, Lock S, Thomas J, et al. An analysis of the effect of routine medications on hemodialysis vascular access survival. Nephron. 1998;**78**(3): 365-368

[108] Chen FA, Chien CC, Chen YW, Wu YT, Lin CC. Angiotensin converting-enzyme inhibitors, angiotensin receptor blockers, and calcium channel blockers are associated with prolonged vascular access patency in uremic patients undergoing hemodialysis. PLoS One. 2016;**11**(11): e0166362

[109] Taber TE, Maikranz PS, Haag BW, Gaylord GM, Dilley RS, Ehrman KO, et al. Maintenance of adequate hemodialysis access. Prevention of neointimal hyperplasia. ASAIO Journal. 1995;**41**(4):842-846

[110] Huang P, Hawthorne WJ, Peng A, Angeli GL, Medbury HJ, Fletcher JP. Calcium channel antagonist verapamil inhibits neointimal formation and enhances apoptosis in a vascular graft model. American Journal of Surgery. 2001;**181**(6):492-498

[111] Bashar K, Zafar A, Elsheikh S, Healy DA, Clarke-Moloney M, Casserly L, et al. Predictive parameters of arteriovenous fistula functional maturation in a population of patients with end-stage renal disease. PLoS One. 2015;**10**(3):e0119958

[112] Doi S, Masaki T, Shigemoto K, Harada S, Yorioka N. Calcium channel antagonists reduce restenosis after percutaneous transluminal angioplasty of an arteriovenous fistula in hemodialysis patients. Therapeutic Apheresis and Dialysis. 2008;**12**(3): 232-236

[113] Manson RJ, Ebner A, Gallo S, Chemla E, Mantell M, Deaton D, et al. Arteriovenous fistula creation using the optiflow vascular anastomosis device: A first in man pilot study. Seminars in Dialysis. 2013;**26**(1):97-99

[114] Lok CE, Rajan DK, Clement J, Kiaii M, Sidhu R, Thomson K, et al. Endovascular proximal forearm arteriovenous fistula for hemodialysis access: Results of the prospective, multicenter Novel Endovascular Access Trial (NEAT). American Journal of Kidney Diseases. 2017;**70**(4):486-497

[115] Lin CC, Yang WC, Chen MC, Liu WS, Yang CY, Lee PC. Effect of far infrared therapy on arteriovenous fistula maturation: An open-label randomized controlled trial. American Journal of Kidney Diseases. 2013;**62**(2): 304-311

[116] Lin CC, Chang CF, Lai MY, Chen TW, Lee PC, Yang WC. Far-infrared therapy: A novel treatment to improve access blood flow and unassisted patency of arteriovenous fistula in hemodialysis patients. Journal of the American Society of Nephrology. 2007; **18**(3):985-992

[117] Hye RJ, Peden EK, O'Connor TP, Browne BJ, Dixon BS, Schanzer AS, et al. Human type I pancreatic elastase treatment of arteriovenous fistulas in patients with chronic kidney disease. Journal of Vascular Surgery. 2014;**60**(2): 454-461 e1

[118] Dwivedi AJ, Roy-Chaudhury P, Peden EK, Browne BJ, Ladenheim ED, Scavo VA, et al. Application of human type I pancreatic elastase (PRT-201) to

the venous anastomosis of arteriovenous grafts in patients with chronic kidney disease. The Journal of Vascular Access. 2014;**15**(5):376-384

[119] Nugent HM, Sjin RT, White D, Milton LG, Manson RJ, Lawson JH, et al. Adventitial endothelial implants reduce matrix metalloproteinase-2 expression and increase luminal diameter in porcine arteriovenous grafts. Journal of Vascular Surgery. 2007;**46**(3):548-556

[120] Nugent HM, Groothuis A, Seifert P, Guerraro JL, Nedelman M, Mohanakumar T, et al. Perivascular endothelial implants inhibit intimal hyperplasia in a model of arteriovenous fistulae: A safety and efficacy study in the pig. Journal of Vascular Research. 2002;**39**(6):524-533

[121] Conte MS, Nugent HM, Gaccione P, Guleria I, Roy-Chaudhury P, Lawson JH. Multicenter phase I/II trial of the safety of allogeneic endothelial cell implants after the creation of arteriovenous access for hemodialysis use: The V-HEALTH study. Journal of Vascular Surgery. 2009; **50**(6):1359-1368 e1

[122] Paulson WD, Kipshidze N, Kipiani K, Beridze N, DeVita MV, Shenoy S, et al. Safety and efficacy of local periadventitial delivery of sirolimus for improving hemodialysis graft patency: First human experience with a sirolimus-eluting collagen membrane (Coll-R). Nephrology, Dialysis, Transplantation. 2012;**27**(3):1219-1224

[123] Kitrou PM, Spiliopoulos S, Katsanos K, Papachristou E, Siablis D, Karnabatidis D. Paclitaxel-coated versus plain balloon angioplasty for dysfunctional arteriovenous fistulae: One-year results of a prospective randomized controlled trial. Journal of Vascular and Interventional Radiology. 2015;**26**(3):348-354

[124] Katsanos K, Karnabatidis D, Kitrou P, Spiliopoulos S, Christeas N, Siablis D. Paclitaxel-coated balloon angioplasty vs. plain balloon dilation for the treatment of failing dialysis access: 6-month interim results from a prospective randomized controlled trial. Journal of Endovascular Therapy. 2012;**19**(2): 263-272

[125] Remuzzi A, Ene-Iordache B. Novel paradigms for dialysis vascular access: Upstream hemodynamics and vascular remodeling in dialysis access stenosis. Clinical Journal of the American Society of Nephrology. 2013;**8**(12): 2186-2193

[126] Bharat A, Jaenicke M, Shenoy S. A novel technique of vascular anastomosis to prevent juxta-anastomotic stenosis following arteriovenous fistula creation. Journal of Vascular Surgery. 2012;**55**(1): 274-280

[127] Chemla E, Tavakoli A, Nikam M, Mitra S, Malete T, Evans J, et al. Arteriovenous fistula creation using the Optiflow vascular anastomotic connector: The OPEN (Optiflow PatEncy and MaturatioN) study. The Journal of Vascular Access. 2014;**15**(1): 38-44

[128] Lee T, Roy-Chaudhury P. Advances and new frontiers in the pathophysiology of venous neointimal hyperplasia and dialysis access stenosis. Advances in Chronic Kidney Disease. 2009;**16**(5):329-338

[129] Hartel M, Hoffmann G, Wente MN, Martignoni ME, Buchler MW, Friess H. Randomized clinical trial of the influence of local water-filtered infrared A irradiation on wound healing after abdominal surgery. The British Journal of Surgery. 2006;**93**(8):952-960

[130] Imamura M, Biro S, Kihara T, Yoshifuku S, Takasaki K, Otsuji Y, et al. Repeated thermal therapy improves impaired vascular endothelial function in patients with coronary risk factors. Journal of the American College of Cardiology. 2001;**38**(4): 1083-1088

[131] Wan Q, Yang S, Li L, Chu F. Effects of far infrared therapy on arteriovenous fistulas in hemodialysis patients: A meta-analysis. Renal Failure. 2017;**39**(1):613-622

[132] Dobrin PB, Canfield TR. Elastase, collagenase, and the biaxial elastic properties of dog carotid artery. The American Journal of Physiology. 1984; **247**(1 Pt 2):H124-H131

[133] Tani T, Kawashima I, Furukawa H, Ohmine T, Takiguchi Y. Characterization of a silent gene for human pancreatic elastase I: Structure of the 5′-flanking region. Journal of Biochemistry. 1987;**101**(3):591-599

[134] Talas U, Dunlop J, Khalaf S, Leigh IM, Kelsell DP. Human elastase 1: Evidence for expression in the skin and the identification of a frequent frameshift polymorphism. The Journal of Investigative Dermatology. 2000; **114**(1):165-170

[135] Peden EK, Leeser DB, Dixon BS, El-Khatib MT, Roy-Chaudhury P, Lawson JH, et al. A multi-center, dose-escalation study of human type I pancreatic elastase (PRT-201) administered after arteriovenous fistula creation. The Journal of Vascular Access. 2013;**14**(2): 143-151

[136] Qamar AA, Burke SK, Lafleur JD, Ding BC, Bland KS, Wong MD, et al. The ability of serum from alpha 1-antitrypsin-deficient patients to inhibit PRT-201, a recombinant human type I pancreatic elastase. Biotechnology and Applied Biochemistry. 2012;**59**(1): 22-28

[137] Hance K, Franano F, Henry C. Prot-101 dilates AV fistula (AVF) outflow veins and reduces intimal hyperplasia in a rabbit model. Journal of the American Society of Nephrology. 2005;**16**:11A

[138] Franano FN, Hance K, Bland K, Burke S. PRT-201 dilates outflow veins and improves maturation rates in a rabbit model of AVF. In: Nephrology Dialysis Transplantation. Oxford, England: Oxford Univ Press; 2007

[139] Charron T, Nili N, Strauss BH. The cell cycle: A critical therapeutic target to prevent vascular proliferative disease. The Canadian Journal of Cardiology. 2006;**22**(Suppl B):41B-55B

[140] Zhu W, Masaki T, Cheung AK, Kern SE. In-vitro release of Rapamycin from a thermosensitive polymer for the inhibition of vascular smooth muscle cell proliferation. Journal of Bioequivalence and Bioavailability. 2009;**1**:3-12

[141] Morice MC, Serruys PW, Barragan P, Bode C, Van Es GA, Stoll HP, et al. Long-term clinical outcomes with sirolimus-eluting coronary stents: Five-year results of the RAVEL trial. Journal of the American College of Cardiology. 2007;**50**(14):1299-1304

[142] Yachi S, Tanabe K, Tanimoto S, Aoki J, Nakazawa G, Yamamoto H, et al. Clinical and angiographic outcomes following percutaneous coronary intervention with sirolimus-eluting stents versus bare-metal stents in hemodialysis patients. American Journal of Kidney Diseases. 2009;**54**(2):299-306

[143] Weisz G, Leon MB, Holmes DR Jr, Kereiakes DJ, Popma JJ, Teirstein PS, et al. Five-year follow-up after sirolimus-eluting stent implantation results of the SIRIUS (Sirolimus-Eluting Stent in De-Novo Native Coronary Lesions) trial. Journal of the American College of Cardiology. 2009;**53**(17): 1488-1497

[144] Roy-Chaudhury P, Kruska L. Future directions for vascular access for hemodialysis. Seminars in Dialysis. 2015;**28**(2):107-113

[145] Scheller B, Hehrlein C, Bocksch W, Rutsch W, Haghi D, Dietz U, et al. Treatment of coronary in-stent

restenosis with a paclitaxel-coated balloon catheter. The New England Journal of Medicine. 2006;**355**(20): 2113-2124

[146] Tepe G, Zeller T, Albrecht T, Heller S, Schwarzwalder U, Beregi JP, et al. Local delivery of paclitaxel to inhibit restenosis during angioplasty of the leg. The New England Journal of Medicine. 2008;**358**(7):689-699

[147] Lai CC, Fang HC, Tseng CJ, Liu CP, Mar GY. Percutaneous angioplasty using a paclitaxel-coated balloon improves target lesion restenosis on inflow lesions of autogenous radiocephalic fistulas: A pilot study. Journal of Vascular and Interventional Radiology. 2014;**25**(4): 535-541

[148] Allon M, Bailey R, Ballard R, Deierhoi MH, Hamrick K, Oser R, et al. A multidisciplinary approach to hemodialysis access: Prospective evaluation. Kidney International. 1998; **53**(2):473-479

[149] Arora P, Obrador GT, Ruthazer R, KAUSZ AT, Meyer KB, Jenuleson CS, et al. Prevalence, predictors, and consequences of late nephrology referral at a tertiary care center. Journal of the American Society of Nephrology. 1999; **10**(6):1281-1286

[150] Roubicek C, Brunet P, Huiart L, Thirion X, Leonetti F, Dussol B, et al. Timing of nephrology referral: Influence on mortality and morbidity. American Journal of Kidney Diseases. 2000;**36**(1): 35-41

[151] Dwyer A, Shelton P, Brier M, Aronoff G. A vascular access coordinator improves the prevalent fistula rate. Seminars in Dialysis. 2012; **25**(2):239-243

[152] Silva MB Jr, Hobson II RW, Pappas PJ, Jamil Z, Araki CT, Goldberg MC, et al. A strategy for increasing use of autogenous hemodialysis access procedures: Impact of preoperative noninvasive evaluation. Journal of Vascular Surgery. 1998;**27**(2):302-308

[153] Robbin ML, Gallichio MH, Deierhoi MH, Young CJ, Weber TM, Allon M. US vascular mapping before hemodialysis access placement. Radiology. 2000;**217**(1):83-88

[154] Allon M, Lockhart ME, Lilly RZ, Gallichio MH, Young CJ, Barker J, et al. Effect of preoperative sonographic mapping on vascular access outcomes in hemodialysis patients. Kidney International. 2001;**60**(5):2013-2020

Section 5

Risk Stratification in Vascular Access

Chapter 5

Promising Role of Vascular Endothelial Growth Factor-A in Risk Stratification after PCI

Olga V. Petyunina, Mykola P. Kopytsya, Iurii S. Rudyk and Ganna S. Isayeva

Abstract

Vascular endothelial growth factor-A (VEGF-A), dimeric glycoprotein, is a potent endothelial cell-specific mitogen which plays a key role in angiogenesis, especially in response to ischemia. Biomarkers reflect various pathophysiological faces of spherical LV transformation that related to myocardial stress due to persisted ischemia, fibrosis, and inflammation, and they may be helpful to improve risk stratification, more personalized medical approach for creating of individual medical care for HF preventing and adjusted treatment after STEMI. VEGF-A decrease ≤172.4 pg./ml on the 7th day of STEMI allows to prognose after infarction angina after 6-month observation (area under curve (AUC) 0.697, with sensitivity 88.9% and specificity 50.9%; 95% CI 0.567–0.807, P = 0.0515). Anxiety and depression 10–14 days before MI associated with VEGF-A level decrease (anxiety (Taylor): OR 0.834, 95% CI 0.726–0.959, P = 0.0107; depression (HADS): OR 0.741, 95% CI 0.535–1.027, P = 0.0519. Cut-off VEGF-A level ≤201.86 pg./ml on the 7th day of STEMI (AUC 0.711, sensitivity 85.7% and specificity 57.9%; 95% CI 0.513–0.908, P = 0.036) was effective for prognosis of dysadaptive left ventricular remodeling in STEMI patients after 6-month observation period. These findings may open new approach to stratify patients with successful coronary revascularization at risk of HF.

Keywords: vascular endothelial growth factor-A, STEMI, prognostication

1. Introduction

Vascular endothelial growth factor-A (VEGF-A) plays a key role in inducing angiogenesis. Angiogenesis is a multifunctional process of new vessels formation by gemmation or by cleavage of the already existing ones. There are the following successive stages of angiogenesis: (1) vasodilatation; (2) migration with adhesion and proliferation of endothelial cells; (3) formation of the vascular wall of a new three-layer vascular tube that develops as the circulation restores [1]. The VEGF was discovered in 1983 [2] as a factor raising vascular permeability, further evidence of a wider range of cytokine activity was obtained. There are 7 representatives of the VEGF family—VEGF-A, B, C, D, E, F, the growth factor of the placenta. The most common is VEGF-A, which is a homodimeric highly glycosylated protein with the molecular weight of 36–46 kDa. VEGF is registered in the heart, lungs, kidneys, adrenal glands, liver, spleen, stomach, and expression of the protein grows under the pathology conditions. VEGF-A is represented by homodimeric isoforms consisting of 121, 145, 148, 165, 183, 189, 206 amino acid residues, among which the essential for the vascular system adequate development is VEGF-165 [3–6].

VEGF-A is produced by endothelial cells, smooth muscle vessels, macrophages, cardiac fibroblasts, lymphocytes, polymorphous nuclear cells, megakaryocytes, monocytes, platelets. Expression of VEGF-A depends on hypoxia, including hypoxia-induced factor, proangiogenic factors (HIF-1, EGF, PDGF, FGF, IL-1-beta), angiotensin II, endotoxin, high glucose level, IL-6, IL-8, IL-10, pH of the medium, oxygen concentration [4–6]. Its products are enhanced by aggregation of platelets, stretching of the left ventricle myocardium. VEGF is a proinflammatory cytokine, it inhibits the formation of dendritic cells, promotes the expression of monocytes, macrophages, leukocytes migration, stimulates adhesive molecules, and the activity of CD34 [7].

VEGF-A is a promoter of the collaterals formation in the ischemic myocardium, has a positive effect on revascularization through the following mechanisms: selective mitogenic effect on endothelial cells, stimulation of vascular endothelial cells expression, their proliferation, regeneration, vascular permeability increase, vasodilatation by activating NO synthase and prostacyclin, inhibition of apoptosis, matrix proteinase products. VEGF has antithrombotic properties due to the activation of serine proteases, urokinase, plasminogen activator, and the thrombolytic enzymes generation. However, VEGF induces the formation of the Willebrand factor and thrombogenesis [3, 4, 7].

In coronary artery disease (CAD), the double role of VEGF-A has been determined: under the conditions of acute or chronic myocardial ischemia, VEGF-A is a promoter of the coronary collaterals development, which promotes adequate blood circulation, oxygen saturation, cardiomyocyte loss prevention, heart remodeling improvement, and ultimately, a positive cardioprotective effect [8–11]. However, the negative component of the VEGF-A is its proatherogenic properties [12], which are implemented through the protein participation in the inflammatory infiltration of the atherosclerotic plaque, its neovascularization and destabilization. The VEGF expression promotes the process of monocytes migration with subsequent transformation into macrophages, the formation of foam cells and atherosclerotic tissues. The VEGF stimulates the matrix metalloprotease expression, which causes the extracellular matrix dissolution and the endothelium migration into a collagen gel with the endothelial tubes formation. The de novo formed vessels contribute to the plaque growth, its rupture, and destabilization of the clinical course in coronary artery disease [7, 13].

Information on changes in the VEGF-A level with stable CAD compared to the healthy group varied from its increase [14–16], to decrease [17] or lack of changes [18]. A number of studies have shown a direct correlation between the level of VEGF-A growth and the degree of damage to coronary vessels. Kucukardali et al. [16], examined the relationship in patients with proven CHD between the level of VEGF-A in blood plasma and the degree of coronary occlusion and the traditional risk factors. Groups with normal coronary angiogram (control), critical coronary injuries (with stenosis >70%) and non-critical changes (with stenosis of 40–70%) were selected. Logistic regression analysis showed that the VEGF-A level in patients with critical coronary sclerosis was significantly higher than in patients with normal coronary angiogram and non-critical stenosis. Higher levels of total cholesterol and LDL cholesterol in patients with critical stenosis were detected, VEGF-A negative correlation with hemoglobin and the positive correlation between VEGF-A and the age. No relationship was found between VEGF-A and other cardiac risk factors. The authors believe that the VEGF-A level growth in patients with coronary heart disease indicates critical coronary sclerosis [16]. Lin et al. [14], showed that the

VEGF-A level in patients with total coronary occlusion was higher than in patients with partial stenotic injuries, indicating the compensatory role of the VEGF-A in angiogenesis. Nakajama et al. [15], in patients with marked coronary atherosclerosis, detected increased levels of VEGF-A compared to moderate stenosis or its lack thereof. Alber et al. [18], however, did not find correlations between the concentration of VEGF-A in the blood plasma, the presence, severity and extent of coronary vessels injuries. The authors drew attention to the fact that in patients treated with statins, the level of VEGF-A was lower, this trend indicates the mechanisms of statins' antiangiogenic effect.

Ramos et al. [17], studied the dynamics of the VEGF-A level after PCI and its role as a predictor of major adverse cardiovascular events (MACE). Patients with ACS (STEMI, MI without ST segment elevation, unstable angina) and without ACS with stable angina pectoris were examined. The content of VEGF-A in the blood serum before PCI did not depend on the clinical form and was lower than that in the healthy group. The level of VEGF-A grew 1 month after revascularization and remained stable during 1 year of observation, reaching the control group's value. The results indicate the positive role of the VEGF-A level growth in the endothelium regeneration.

Angiogenesis and the coronary collaterals formation in AMI is of particular importance as an adaptation process in response to myocardial hypoxia. An increase in collateral circulation limits myocardial ischemia, prevents the spread of necrosis, improves the function of the myocardium [8]. The ability of VEGF-A to promote the development of collateral circulation has been demonstrated on the MI experimental models in animals. The use of VEGF for therapeutic angiogenesis in AMI in experimental animals was performed by intracardiac administration of VEGF-encoding genes, use of deproteinized isoforms of DNA (pVEGF 165), adenoviral vectors (Ad VEGF 121), etc. As a result, initially, in the perinecrotic zone, in remote areas, and then in the MI zone, there was an increase in the number of functioning capillaries, their bulk surface, anastomoses, activation of capillary collateral circulation [1, 9], improvement of cardiac micro vessels regeneration, cardiac function [10], fibrosis reduction and increasing of the myocardium contractile function [11], which ultimately reflects the cardioprotective effects of VEGF-A as a result of angiogenesis and endothelial cells proliferation.

In most clinical studies, an increase in the VEGF-A level in AMI compared to healthy persons, patients with stable or unstable angina [8, 19–24] was determined. At the same time, in works by Ramos et al. [17], the level of VEGF-A in patients with CAD was lower than in healthy persons, and its differences between clinical forms of coronary heart disease were not found.

The analysis of the factors influencing the VEGF level growth in AMI showed the following. The classic cardiovascular risk factors (gender, age, hypertension, overweight, diabetes mellitus, smoking, hypercholesterolemia) in patients with AMI did not correlate with the VEGF-A level [8, 17, 21, 25], although the VEGF-A level in patients with H, DM, high BMI, obesity, HF without MI were different from healthy ones.

Comparison of the VEGF-A level in patients with AMI with single- and multi-vascular coronary sclerosis revealed a lack of cytokine correlation with a heart attack-dependent coronary artery [8, 21, 26], simultaneously, Wojakovski et al. [24], determined higher values of VEGF-A in the blood serum in patients with MI with multi-vessel injuries compared to those with single-vessel ones. No relationship was found between the VEGF level and the heart attack localization [8]. Results of the connection between the VEGF and the size of the myocardial injury, which were determined by the level of CK, CK-MB cardiomarkers, were ambiguous. Kranz et al. [8], Shimokawahara et al. [21] did not find any connection between

VEGF-A and CK; Hojo et al. [20], Ogawa et al. [22], showed a positive correlation between VEGF-A and CK-MB and suggested an association between the prevalence of MI and the increase in the VEGF-A formation.

Several studies were devoted to the dynamics of VEGF-A in the acute phase of the MI and the subsequent post-infarction prognosis. The VEGF-A level in AMI after PCI peaked on the 7th–14th days [8, 20, 21, 27, 28] and returned to the norm for 6 months [28]. According to experimental data, administering of VEGF 124 before the coronary artery occlusion was accompanied by a pronounced activation of the angiogenesis process, collateral circulation in the perinecrotic zone and the distant regions of myocardium on the 7th day of the experiment [1]. It is possible to assume that a peak increase in the VEGF-A level for 7–10 days of AMI corresponds to the beginning of active angiogenesis. Mechanisms of VEGF-A endogenous expression activation in AMI are associated with response to hypoxia and acute myocardial ischemia and are implemented at the molecular level. A number of studies have provided additional information on the pathogenesis of VEGF-A expression enhancement in AMI. Thus, according to Hojo et al. [20], in patients with AMI, VEGF-A level was determined in the blood serum and in mononuclear cells of peripheral blood. Its blood serum levels peaked at the 14th day of AMI and correlated positively with the CK. There was a slight difference in the VEGF-A level in mononuclear cells: it was maximally elevated on the 7th day of AMI, did not correlate with CK, its reliably higher values were determined in patients with LVEF—≥40% compared to the VEGF group <40%. The authors believe that peripheral blood mononuclear cells are an important source of VEGF-A, and if they are mononuclear cells that infiltrate myocardium injured by infarction, VEGF-A, locally formed by mononuclear cells, promotes endothelial proliferation, the formation of microvessels, recovery of the damaged endothelium, healing of the infarcted myocardium, performing an important role in improving systolic function after MI [20].

Kranz et al. [8], observed a significant increase in the level of VEGF-A in the blood of AMI patients, which was maximally expressed on the 7th–10th days and reached the baseline value for 6 months, with unstable angina, the cytokine value did not reliably differ from the control. The absence of VEGF-A level differences in the blood serum and coronary sinus was detected unexpectedly, i.e. the infracted myocardium is not the main source of VEGF-A in the blood stream. The authors found a reliable growth in the number of platelets in the dynamics of MI. Platelets are an important source of VEGF-A, and the cytokine level growth in AMI can be explained by an increase in the number of platelets, and their aggregation enhancement, which leads to the secretion of growth factors from alpha granules.

Korybalska et al. [23], determined a significant increase in the level of VEGF-A in the blood serum of STEMI patients compared to healthy individuals. The number of platelets did not differ between patients with STEMI and healthy persons, however, in patients with STEMI, a direct reliable correlation between VEGF-A and platelets was found. The cytokine concentration increased immediately after retrosternal pain onset in patients with occlusive thrombi, which corresponded to the 3–4° by the TIMI scale. The authors believe that the VEGF-A level growth in patients with STEMI occurs not only due to ischemia and hypoxia of the myocardium, but can also be formed from activated platelets and characterize patients with increased intracoronary thrombosis [23].

Wojakovski et al. [24], studied the correlation between the levels of the VEGF, pro- and anti-inflammatory markers, traditional risk factors, the status of systolic function of the lungs, and the marker of inflammation—high sensitive CRP (hsCRP) in patients with AMI and stable angina. The authors found that the level of VEGF-A in patients with AMI was reliably higher than in those with stable angina, in AMI patients with a multi-vessel injury it was higher than in those with mono-vascular injury, in group with EF <40% and Killip III–IV class in comparison with EF >40% and Killip I–II class, with a duration of pain syndrome >6 h compared to that of <6 h. Acute myocardial ischemia was associated with a reduction in the level of anti-inflammatory cytokine IL-10. Although the authors did not find correlation between VEGF-A and IL-10, they believe that changes of these cytokines concentration will help identify persons with high cardiovascular risk. The level of hsCRP, a marker, the importance of which was proven in inflammation, had a negative correlation with anti-inflammatory cytokine IL-10 and a positive one with VEGF-A, which indicates the VEGF-A participation in the immune response to AMI.

Eržen et al. [28], determined a reliable increase in the level of the VEGF in patients with MI, on average 20.5 months ago, compared to the control, a reliable positive correlation between the VEGF level and the pro-inflammatory IL-6 and IL-8 molecules, lack of correlation between VEGF and the atherosclerotic injury parameters, although dilatation of the right shoulder artery and the intima-media thickness of the common carotid artery in the examined patients were significantly weakened. The authors believe that the VEGF-A increase in the stable phase after the past MI is a part of inflammatory activity, since VEGF-A in these patients stimulates neovascularization, inflammation of the plaque and promotes its destabilization, its level increase may have a negative prognostic value.

An important component in raising the VEGF-A level, angiogenesis enhancing, cardiac blood flow, myocardial perfusion, oxygen transport, and the entry of energy substrates into cardiomyocytes is its effect on the structural and functional parameters of the myocardium, followed by adaptive or dysadaptive remodeling. Moreover, the VEGF-A expression and its receptors in cardiac fibroblasts and non-endothelial cells with properties of fibroblasts that perform tissue growth and regeneration assumes cytokine involvement in the process of myocardial remodeling in the ischemia and necrosis zones [29]. With experimental MI in rats, administration of VEGF-A-165 and VEGF-B-167 into the myocardium reduced myocardial fibrosis and improved its contractile function, viability, and remodeling of the left ventricle [11]. Administration of anti-P-selectin-conjugated liposomes containing the VEGF to experimental MI rats was accompanied by a 37% reduction in collagen deposition in the myocardium, a significant improvement in the pressure of the LV filling, with a significant improvement in the cardiac function 4 weeks after the MI: LV EDD reduction, growth of the fractional shortening, at the same time, the number of anatomical and perfused vessels increased [10, 30, 31]. Injection of the collagen-bound VEGF domain resulted in the infarction area reduction, improvement of the processes of LV remodeling within 3 months, and 12 months later, in the MI zone, mature vasculature and myocardium-like tissues were observed. Thus, the protection of cardiomyocytes from apoptosis and involvement of precursor cells in the infarction zone occurred [32].

The results of clinical studies on the correlation between VEGF-A and post-infarction remodeling are ambiguous. Thus, in the AMI patients, the indices of LV volumes, determined by ventriculography on the 14th day of AMI, were increased in the group with a high peak VEGF-A value compared to the low VEGF-A value group, the peak of the VEGF-A plasma level positively correlated with LV EDV and LV ESV. These differences were absent in the chronic phase of MI. The authors believe that endogenous VEGF-A plays an important role in the dilatation of LV in patients with AMI [21]. Soeki et al. [33], referred patients, in whom 3 months after the AMI an increase in the EDV-index was more than 5 ml/m^2, to the group with remodeling; the authors did not find changes in the VEGF level between patients with and without remodeling. However, patients with AMI and improvement of systolic function, compared to patients without such improvement, had higher VEGF-A levels in mononuclear cells of the peripheral blood; the authors believe that

VEGF-A, which is formed in mononuclear cells infiltrating the infarcted myocardium, plays an important role in angiogenesis, re-endothelialization, restoration of the LV systolic function after the AMI [20]. Devaux et al. [19], determined the LV remodeling according to the EDV dynamics in the period between the patient's hospitalization and 6 months after the MI; the first group consisted of patients with ΔEDV, which did not undergo significant changes or was decreasing; group 2 included patients whose ΔEDV was increasing. The level of VEGF-B was 69% higher in patients with $\Delta EDV \leq 0$ than in patients with $\Delta EDV > 0$. The authors believe that the low level of VEGF-B in blood with AMI is associated with a high risk of LV remodeling and is its predictor.

In accordance with the spectrum of the VEGF biological cardiovascular effects, a number of studies are devoted to the role of cytokine for the long-term prognosis in patients with MI. The contradictory results were obtained. Thus, Heeschen et al. [34], determined the level of VEGF-A in plasma of 1090 patients with ACS 8.7 h after the onset of the event. The frequency of major cardiovascular complications during the 6 months of observation was high in patients with the initially increased VEGF-A level. But other studies have obtained evidence that it is the decrease in the VEGF-A level which is an independent prognostic factor of recurrent cardiovascular events in other studies. Thus, Niu et al. [25], determined the VEGF-A level on the 7th day after MI, groups with low and high (less than or greater than 190 ng/ml) median VEGF-A levels. Repeated examinations were carried out every 2 months during the year; MACE, which included cardiovascular death, heart failure, severe arrhythmias, cardiogenic shock and post-infarction angina, were recorded. Within 6 months, the MACE frequency in the VEGF-A high-level group was significantly lower than in the low-cytokine group. Accordingly, the VEGF-A concentration in the group of patients without MACE was significantly higher than that in the MACE group.

Multivariant regression analysis showed that the decrease of the VEGF-A level is an independent MACE risk factor, its high value on the 7th day after AMI determines a positive long-term prognosis. Matsudaira et al. [27], examined 879 patients with AMI after successful PCI within the framework of a prospective, multicenter NAMIS study (Nagoya Acute Myocardial Infarction Study). According to VEGF-A level terciles, which was determined on the 7th day of AMI, 3 groups were formed, in which within 6 months of observation the major unfavorable cardiac and cerebral events were determined: cardiac death, repeated ACS, hospitalization for heart failure, strokes. Compared to the "medium" tercile, patients with the "low" tercile had a much higher risk of MACE. The authors believe that the low of VEGF-A level on the 7th day after AMI is associated with a significant increase in the MACE risk for 6 months.

Unlike the previous authors, Ramos et al. [17], determined that the level of VEGF-A in patients with AMI was lower than that of healthy individuals at admission, it was getting increased within 1 month term and remained steadily increased up to 1 year of observation. But in this study, it was shown that a decrease in the VEGF-A level < 40.8 pg./ml contributed to an increased risk of MACE for 5 years. The obtained results indicated the positive role of VEGF-A in the cardiovascular circulation restoration and confirmed its prognostic importance. In studies of Teplyakov et al. [35], the degree of ischemic genesis cardiac failure progression, most of the examined were postinfarction patients, there was a decrease in the VEGF-A level, and the initial low VEGF-A level characterized the unfavorable CHF course.

It is known that psychological stress is involved in the development and progression of cardiovascular disease. Thus, in an INTERHEART study performed in 52 world countries, anxiety and depression ranked third among the MI risk factors [36]. In Surtees et al. [37], within the 8.5 years period of observation, patients with a "major" depression were by 2.7 times more likely to die from the coronary heart disease. Findings from this large prospective cohort study suggest that increased psychological distress is associated with elevated stroke risk. Episodic major depressive disorder was not associated with incident stroke in this study. Doering et al. [38], demonstrated that the presence of anxiety and depression was the predictor of the overall death-rate in patients with coronary artery disease. Versteeg et al. [39], showed that depression was independently associated with an increased risk of the overall death-rate for 5 years in patients with coronary artery disease. In the study by Beach et al. [40], the high level of depression by the Patient Health Questionaire-9 (PHQ-9) was reliably associated with re-hospitalization after 6 months in patients with acute coronary syndrome, heart failure, or arrhythmia.

Mechanisms to be associated with anxiety-depressive disorders (ADD) and cardiovascular diseases are complex and take into account both behavioral and physiological factors: smoking, lifestyle underactivity, obesity, as well as increased platelet aggregation, arterial pressure, reduced insulin sensitivity and disordered endothelial function [41, 42].

In recent years, the evidence base for participation of VEGF-A in the cerebrovascular disease pathogenesis, including ADD, is growing. VEGF-A is known to be involved in such processes in the central nervous system as the ontogenetic development of the nervous system, which includes the processes of migration, differentiation, synaptogenesis, myelination, neuroprotection, stimulation of neurogenesis in adulthood, post-ischemic restoration of cerebral and vessel tissues, stimulation of memory formation mechanisms. VEGF-A participates in all phases of neuro-and angiogenesis: formation of blood vessels de-novo from mesenchymal stem cells, formation of new capillaries, expansion of arteriolar anastomoses, and also demonstrates direct neurotrophic and neuroprotective properties. Thus, the role of VEGF in the pathogenesis of cerebrovascular pathology, including anxiety-depressive disorders, is to combine angiotropic and neurotropic activity [43].

An increase in the VEGF-A level in patients with major depression was observed [44–48]; the correlation between depression and VEGF-A is confirmed by the fact that cytokine stimulates neurogenesis caused by antidepressants [49, 50]. In patients with coronary heart disease, higher levels of VEGF-A, CRP, IL-6 gene expression and cortisol level reduction were detected, indicating an increase in immune-mediated activity [51].

It should be noted that in these works, patients with major depression were somatically healthy, or patients with coronary artery disease were with a stable course. However, in acute experimental ischemia, psychological stress was associated with a decrease in the VEGF-A and its signaling molecules (P44/P42, MAPK, Akt) expression, violation of neurovascularization at the macro- and microvascular levels, which the authors associate with the oxidative stress activation in the ischemic tissue [52].

The aim of our research was investigation of association between VEGF-A level in STEMI patients with TIMI III and development of repeated coronary events and adverse remodeling within 6-month follow-up and determination of the factors influencing this relationship.

2. Material and methods

2.1 Patients

Sixty-two patients with STEMI, 51 (82.3%) male and 11 (17.7%) female, at the average age (58.63 ± 8.90) years with acute STEMI during 2–12 h of symptoms onset in a given period between 2016 and 2017. STEMI was diagnosed according to ECS Guidelines [53]. Inclusion criteria were: confirmed STEMI, age >18 years old, and lack of contraindication to PCI. Non-inclusion criteria were previous myocardial infarction, established chronic HFrEF, HFmrEF and HFpEF, known malignancy, severe comorbidities (anemia, chronic obstructive lung disease, bronchial asthma, liver cirrhosis, chronic kidney disease, valvular heart disease, bleeding), inability to understand of written informed consent. Control group consisted of 20 persons comparable of age and sex. Patients were hospitalized to the Department of prevention and treatment of emergency conditions of Government institution "L.T. Malaya Therapy National Institute of the National Academy of medical science of Ukraine" after selective coronaroangiography (SCAG) with stenting of infarct-related artery, were performed in the Institute of general and emergency surgery n.a. V.T. Zaitsev. Repeated observation performed after 6 month.

Research was performed due to Helsinki Declaration, the protocol was approved by local ethics committee of GI "National Institute of therapy n.a. L.T.Malaya NAMS Ukraine" (protocol No. 8, 29.08.2016). Informed consent was obtained from each patient.

Conventional coronary angiography was performed using Digital X-Ray system "Integris Allura" (Philips Healthcare, Best, The Netherlands) and managed by radial or femoral vascular access. Coronary arteries were visualized with two-to-three orthogonal projections. In this study the contrast "Ultravist-370" (Baier Pharma GmbH, Germany) and automatic contrast injector were used. Primary PCI with bare-metal stent (COMMANDER, "Alvimedica", Turkey) implantation was performed in 36 patients and 26 patients were previously treated with primary thrombolysis (tenecteplase, alteplase) before admission with followed PCI during 6–12 h after initial STEMI confirmation. Thrombolytic therapy performed by tenecteplase, which dosing was calculated depending on patients weight and was no more than 50 mg or alteplase, or tenecteplase—100 mg. All the patients intook medical therapy in accordance to existing recommendations.

Repeated coronary events (after infarction angina) during 6-month observation period were estimated and diagnosed in 9 (14.5%) patients. Left ventricular remodeling as an end point in 6 months after STEMI were assessed too: adverse remodeling was in 29 patients, adaptive—in 33.

2.2 Methods

SYNTAX score (SS) was used to assess the severity of coronary atherosclerotic lesions and was calculated for all PCI-patients by experienced interventional cardiologist. SS was determined for all coronary lesions >50% diameter stenosis in a vessel >1.5 mm based on SS calculator (www.syntaxscore.com). All the patients were divided by the SS level on 3 subgroups—high SS > 32–2 patients, average SS $22 < n \leq 32$–17, low SS ≤ 22–32.

Echo-CG was performed on "Aplio 500 TUS-A500", Toshiba, with usage of sensor with ultrasound frequency of 3.5 MHz during first 24 h from hospitalization. Left ventricular end diastolic volume (LV EDV), left ventricular end systolic volume (LV ESV), left ventricular end diastolic and end systolic diameters (LV EDD, LV ESD), left ventricular myocardial mass (LVMM), left ventricular ejection fraction (LVEF), diastolic dysfunction—maximal rate of early diastolic filling E (m/s), maximal rate of left atrium diastolic rate A (m/s), their ratio—E/A were estimated. Repeated observation was done after 6-month period. VEGF-A level was assessed on the 7th day of STEMI. Late adverse cardiac remodeling was defined as increased LVEDV (>10% from baseline) and/or LVESV (>10% from baseline) for 6 months after acute STEMI managed by PCI.

Hypercholesterolemia (HCE) was diagnosed if total cholesterol (TC) level was above 5.2 mmol/l, and/or low density lipoprotein cholesterol (LDL) level was above 3.0 mmol/l, and/or level of triglycerides (TG) was above 1.7 mmol/l according to with European Cardiology Society dyslipidemia guideline, 2016. Hypertension was diagnosed if systolic blood pressure (SBP) was >140 mm Hg, and/or diastolic blood pressure (DBP) >90 mm Hg according to European guideline on diagnostics and treatment of arterial hypertension, 2018. Type 2 diabetes mellitus determined according to new ADA statement [54].

The level of anxiety during 10–14 days before STEMI estimated due to Taylor questionnaire. High level of anxiety was consistent with less or equal 14 balls, high level—more than 14 balls. Together with Taylor questionnaire, Heart Anxiety and Depression Scale (HADS) was used to diagnose anxiety and depression: 0–7 balls—low level, 8–10—borderline, 11–21—high.

Troponin I (Tn I) level measuring performed with chemo luminescent immunoassay (Humalyzer 2000, Mannheim, Germany). The TnI level average was 0.5–50 ng/ml. Total creatine kinase (CK) and CK MB-fraction (CK-MB) were analyzed using immunoinhibition method on quantitative immunoassay analyzer Humalyzer 2000 (Mannheim, Germany) according to the manufacturers' recommendations. Total cholesterol (TC), low density lipoprotein (LDL) cholesterol, high density lipoprotein (HDL) cholesterol and triglycerides (TG) were measured direct enzymatic method (Roche P800 analyzer, Basel, Switzerland). The intra-assay and inter-assay coefficients of variation were <5%. Fasting glucose level was measured by a double-antibody sandwich immunoassay (Elecsys 1010 analyzer, F. Hoffmann-La Roche Diagnostics, Mannheim, Germany). The intra-assay and inter-assay coefficients of variation were <5%.

Blood research were done at baseline. VEGF-A level determined by enzyme-linked immunosorbent assay with reactives of IBL INTERNATIONAL GMBH, Germany (standard concentrations diapason 0.0–1000 pg./ml, serum control: low—100–200, high—600–1200 pg./ml) in the laboratory of immune-chemical and molecular-genetic researches of GI "National Institute of therapy n.a. L.T. Malaya NAMS Ukraine". Serum VEGF-A level measured in the 7th day of STEMI: in the main group it was equal 160.33 [83.82–299.62] pg./ml, in the control group—112.30 [75.45–164.65] pg./ml ($P = 0.05$).

2.3 Statistical analyses

Statistical data processing was performed with programs Statistica 8.0 (Stat Soft Inc., USA), median (Me) with upper (UQ) and low quartiles (LQ). Continuous variables are presented as mean ± standard deviation when normally distributed, or median and interquartile range if otherwise. Mann-Whitney U-criterion and Wald-Wolfowitz χ^2- criterion were used for intergroup differences. For all types of analysis, all differences were considered statistically significant with $P < 0.05$. Univariate and multivariate logistic statistical analyses were used. The group with repeated coronary events pointed as 1, without events—0, cut-off point with VEGF-A were found.

3. Results

The first group with repeated coronary events (after infarction angina) represented 9 patients (14.5%), the second group consisted from 53 patients without angina to 6 months after STEMI. Cardiovascular risk factors [sex, age, H, DM, HCE, complicated heredity, anxiety-depressive disorders (ADD)] showed the absence of reliable differences between patients of group 1 and 2. VEGF-A level was significantly less in patients from group 1:83.82 [49.14–162.26] pg./ml versus 194.10 [102.54–327.30] pg./ml accordantly, P = 0.049.

ROC-analysis was performed to find VEGF-A level which prognoses repeated coronary events after 6-month observation after STEMI. Cut-off VEGF-A level ≤ 172.4 pg./ml on the 7th day of index event (area under curve (AUC) 0.697, with sensitivity 88.9% and specificity 50.9%; 95% CI 0.567–0.807, P = 0.0515) was effective for differentiation STEMI patients from those without and with unfavorable prognosis of repeated coronary event—after infarction angina (**Figure 1**).

To identify factors influenced on VEGF-A level, univariate and multivariate logistic analysis were performed. In patients with STEMI was revealed association between anxiety and depression levels increase and VEGF-A level decrease (anxiety (Taylor): OR 0.834, 95% CI 0.726–0.959, P = 0.0107; depression (HADS): OR 0.741, 95% CI 0.535–1.027, P = 0.0519.

ROC-analysis for prognostication of dysadaptive left ventricular remodeling was used. Cut-off VEGF-A level ≤ 201.86 pg./ml on the 7th day of STEMI (area under curve (AUC) 0.711, with sensitivity 85.7% and specificity 57.9%; 95% CI 0.513–0.908, P = 0.036) was effective for unfavorable prognosis of dysadaptive left ventricular remodeling of STEMI patients after 6-month observation period (**Figure 2**).

As a result of our research, we revealed than anxiety and depression 10–14 days before MI associated with VEGF-A level decrease (anxiety (Taylor): OR 0.834, 95% CI 0.726–0.959, P = 0.0107; depression (HADS): OR 0.741, 95% CI 0.535–1.027, P = 0.0519. VEGF-A decrease ≤172.4 pg./ml on the 7th day of STEMI allows to prognose

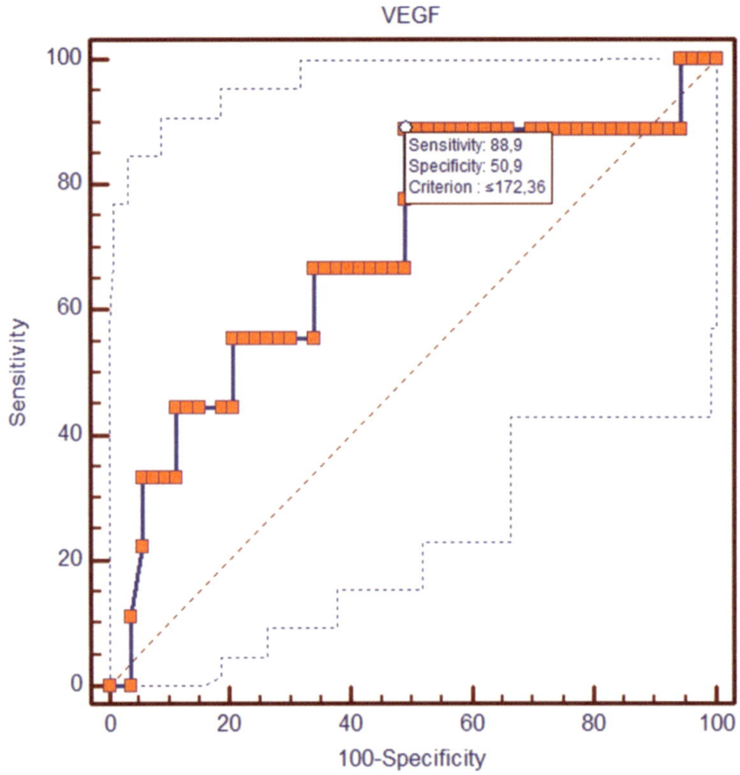

Figure 1.
Cut-off VEGF-A level ≤ 172.4 pg./ml on the 7th day of STEMI (area under curve (AUC) 0.697, with sensitivity 88.9% and specificity 50.9%; 95% CI 0.567–0.807, P = 0.0515) was effective for differentiation STEMI patients from those without and with unfavorable prognosis of repeated coronary event (after infarction angina after 6-month observation).

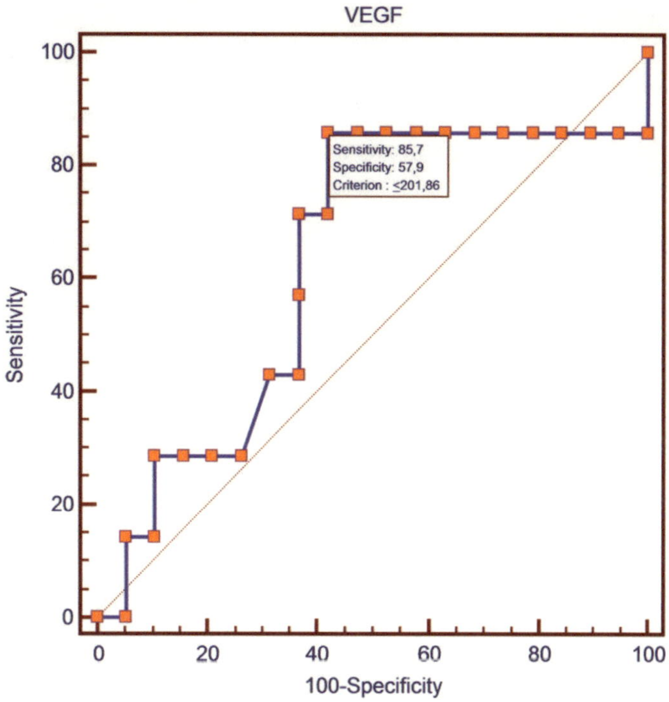

Figure 2.
Cut-off VEGF-A level ≤ 201.86 pg./ml on the 7th day of STEMI (area under curve (AUC) 0.711, with sensitivity 85.7% and specificity 57.9%; 95% CI 0.513–0.908, P = 0.036) was effective for unfavorable prognosis of dysadaptive left ventricular remodeling in STEMI patients after 6-month observation period.

repeated coronary events (after infarction angina) after 6-month observation with sensitivity of 88.9% and specificity 50.9%. Cut-off VEGF-A level ≤ 201.86 pg./ml on the 7th day of STEMI (area under curve (AUC) 0.711, with sensitivity 85.7% and specificity 57.9%; 95% CI 0.513–0.908, P = 0.036) was effective for prognosis of dysadaptive left ventricular remodeling in STEMI patients after 6-month observation period.

4. Conclusion

We have shown that the levels of VEGF-A measured in acute STEMI patients managed by PCI could predict late adverse LV remodeling and after infarction angina. These findings may open new approach to stratify patients with successful coronary revascularization at risk of HF.

Acknowledgements

There are no previous presentations of the information reported in the article. We thank Nataliia Tytarenko and Igor Polivenok for performing ultrasound examination and cardiac interventions respectively. Additionally, we thank, Galina Bugrimenko for her excellent technical assistance. Permission to acknowledge has been obtained.

Conflict of interest

There are no conflicts of interest.

Author contribution

Conception and design: Olga V. Petyunina; writing of the article Olga V. Petyunina, critical revision of the article for intellectual content Mykola P. Kopytsya, Iurii S. Rudyk, Ganna S. Isayeva.

Funding

This research received no specific grant from any funding agency in the public, commercial, or not-for-profit sectors.

Limitation of the study

This was a retrospective observational study and the number of patients was relatively small. A randomized controlled study based on a greater number of patients with a longer observational period is needed to confirm our results.

Founding

The study is a fragment of the research project: "To study the biochemical, genetic mechanisms of reperfusion damage of the myocardium and to assess the cardioprotective effect of antiplatelet therapy in acute myocardial infarction", State Registration No. 0117 U003028.

Author details

Olga V. Petyunina*, Mykola P. Kopytsya, Iurii S. Rudyk and Ganna S. Isayeva
Government Institution "L.T. Malaya Therapy National Institute of NAMS of Ukraine", Kharkiv, Ukraine

*Address all correspondence to: o_petyunina@ukr.net

References

[1] Sisakyan AS, Oganyan VA, Semerdzhyan AB, Petrosyan MV, Sisakyan SA, Gurevich MA. Vliyanie faktora angiogeneza na morfofunkcionalnoe sostoyanie miokarda u krys pri eksperimentalnom infarkte miokarda. Rossijskij kardiologicheskij zhurnal—Russian Cardiology journal. 2008;**2**:63-66 (in russ)

[2] Ferrara N, Davis-Smyth T. The biology of vascular endothelial growth factor. Endocrine Reviews. 1997;**18**:527-543

[3] Hoeben A, Landuyt B, Highley MS, et al. Vascular endothelial growth factor and angiogenesis. Pharmacological Reviews. 2004;**56**(4):549-580. DOI: 10.1124/pr.56.4.3

[4] Ferrara N. Binding to the extracellular matrix and proteolytic processing. Two key mechanisms regulating vascular endothelial growth factor action. Molecular Biology of the Cell. 2010;**21**(5):687-690. DOI: 10.1091/mbc.E09-07-0590

[5] Ferrara N. Vascular endothelial growth factor. Arteriosclerosis, Thrombosis, and Vascular Biology. 2009;**29**(6):789-791. DOI: 10.1161/ATVBAHA.108.179663

[6] Starostin IV, Talitskiy KA, Bulkina OS, Parfenova EV. Karpov YuA collateral blood flow in the myocardium: The role of endothelial growth factor. Kardiologiia—Cardiology. 2012;**11**:49-55 (in russ)

[7] Berezin AE. Predicitive role of circulating vascular endothelial growth factor-1 in patients with cardiovascular diseases. Journal of Disease Markers. 2014;**1**(3) id1013

[8] Kranz A, Rau C, Kochs M, et al. Elevation of vascular endothelial growth factor-A serum levels following acute myocardial infarction. Evidence for its origin and functional significance. Journal of Molecular and Cellular Cardiology. 2000;**32**(1):65-72. DOI: 10.1006/jmcc.1999.1062

[9] Sant'Anna RT, Kalil RAT, Moreno P, Anflor LCJ, Correa DLC, Ludwig R, et al. Gene therapy with VEGF 165 for angiogenesis in experimental acute myocardial infarction. Brazilian Journal of Cardiovascular Surgery. 2003. Print version ISSN 0102-7638; On-line version ISSN 1678-9741. DOI: 10.1590/S0102-76382003000200006

[10] Wang B, Cheheltani R, Rosano J, Crabbe DL, Kiani MF. Targeted delivery of VEGF to treat myocardial infarction. Advances in Experimental Medicine and Biology. 2013;**765**:307-314. DOI: 10.1007/978-1-4614-4989-8_43

[11] Zentilin L, Puligadda U, Lionetti V, Zacchigna S, Collesi C, et al. Cardiomyocyte VEGFR-1 activation by VEGF-B induces compensatory hypertrophy and preserves cardiac function after myocardial infarction. The FASEB Journal. 2010;**24**(5):1467-1478. DOI: 10.1096/fj.09-143180 (Epub Dec 17, 2009)

[12] Kimura K, Hashiguchi T, Deguchi T, et al. Serum VEGF—As a prognostic factor of atherosclerosis. Atherosclerosis. 2007;**194**(1):182-188. DOI: 10.1016/j.atherosclerosis.2006.07.025

[13] Moreno P, Purushothaman KR, Fuster V, Echeverri D, Truszczynska E, et al. Plaque neovascularization is increased in ruptured atherosclerotic lesions of human aorta. Circulation. 2004;**110**(14):2032-2038. DOI: 10.1161/01.CIR.0000143233.87854.23 (Epub Sep 2, 2004)

[14] Lin TH, Yen HW, Su HM, Chien WT, Lu YH, Voon WC, et al. Effects

of total coronary artery occlusion on vascular endothieial growth factor and transforming growth factor beta. The Kaohsiung Journal of Medical Sciences. 2005;**21**(10):460-465

[15] Nakajama K, Tabata S, Yamashita T, et al. Plasma vascular endothelial growth factor level is elevated in patients with multivessel coronary artery disease. Clinical Cardiology. 2004;**27**(5):281-286

[16] Kucukardali Y, Aydogly S, Ozmen N, Yonem A, Solmazgul E, Ozyurt M, et al. The relationship between severity of coronary artery disease and plasma level of vascular endothelial growth factor. Cardiovascular Revascularization Medicine. 2008;**9**:66-70. DOI: 10.1016/j.carrev.2007.11.005

[17] Ramos K, Napoleao P, Selas M, et al. Prognostic Value of VEGF in Patients Submitted to Percutaneous Coronary Intervention. Disease Markers. Hindawi Pub Corp; 2014;**2014**:7. Article ID: 135357. https://doi.org/10.1155/2014/135357

[18] Alber HF, Frick M, Dulak J, et al. Vascular endothelial growth factor (VEGF) plasma concentrations in coronary artery disease. Heart. 2005;**91**(3):365-366. DOI: 10.1136/hrt.2003.021311

[19] Devaux Y, Vausort M, Azuaje F, et al. Low levels of vascular endothelial growth factor B predict left ventricular remodeling after acute myocardial infarction. Journal of Cardiac Failure. 2012;**18**(4):330-337. DOI: 10.1016/j.cardfail.2012.01.010

[20] Hojo Y, Ikeda U, Zhu Y, et al. Expression of vascular endothelial growth factor in patients with acute myocardial infarction. Journal of the American College of Cardiology. 2000;**35**(4):968-973

[21] Shimokawahara H, Jougasaki M, Setoguchi M, et al. Relationsheep between vascular endothelial growth factor and left ventricular dimension in patients with acute myocardial infarction. Journal of Cardiology. 2014;**64**(5):360-365. DOI: 10.1016/j.jjcc.2014.02.017

[22] Ogawa H, Suefuji H, Soejma H, et al. Increased blood vascular endothelial growth factor levels in patients with acute myocardial infarction. Cardiology. 2000;**93**(1-2):93-99. DOI: 7008

[23] Korybalska K, Pyda M, Kawka E, et al. Interpretation of elevated serum VEGF concentration in patients with myocardial infarction. Cytokine. 2011;**54**(1):74-78. DOI: 10.1016/j.ijcard.2012.05.103

[24] Wojakovski W, Maslankiewicz K, Ochala A, et al. The pro- and anti-inflammatory markers in patients with acute myocardial infarction and chronic stable angina. International Journal of Molecular Medicine. 2004;**14**(2):317-322. DOI: 10.3892/ijmm.14.2.317

[25] Niu J, Han X, Qi H, et al. Correlation between vascular endothelial growth factor and long-term prognosis in patients with acute myocardial infarction. Experimental and Therapeutic Medicine. 2016;**12**(1):475-479. DOI: 10.3892/etm.2016.3286

[26] Chung NA, Lydakis C, Belgore F, Li-Saw-Hee FL, Blann AD, Lip GY. Angiogenesis, thrombogenesis, endothelial dysfunction and angiographic severity of coronary artery disease. Heart. 2003;**89**(12):1411-1415

[27] Matsudaira K, Maeda K, Okumura N, et al. Impact of low levels of vascular endothelial growth factor after myocardial infarction on 6-month outcome. Resuls from Nagoya Acute Myocardial Infarction Study. Circulation Journal. 2012;**76**:1509-1516. DOI: 10.1253/circj.CJ-11-1127

[28] Eržen B, Šilar M, Šabovic M. Stable phase post-MI patients

have elevated VEGF levels correlated with inflammation markers, but not with atherosclerotic burden. BMS Cardiovascular Disorders. 2014;**14**:166. DOI: 10.1186/1471-2261-14-166

[29] Chintalgattu V, Nair DM, Katwa LC. Cardiac myofibroblasts: A novel source of vascular endothelial growth factor (VEGF) and its receptors Flt-1 and KDR. Journal of Molecular and Cellular Cardiology. 2003;**35**(3):277-286

[30] Rosano JM, Cheheltani R, Wang B, et al. Targeted delivery of VEGF after a myocardial infarction reduces collagen deposition and improves cardiac feunction. Cardiovascular Engineering and Technology. 2012;**3**(2):237-247. DOI: 10.1007/s13239-012-0089-3

[31] Chelentani R, Rosano JM, Wang B, Kiani MF. Targeted VEGF therapy favorably alters collagen deposition and guality after myocardial infarction. The FASEB Journal. 2010;**24**(1). (Published online Apr 1, 2010) – abstract

[32] Shi C, Zhao Y, Yang Y, Chen C, Hou X, Shao J, et al. Collagen-binding VEGF targeting the cardiac extracellular matrix promotes recovery in porcine chronic myocardial infarction. Biomaterials Science. 2018;**6**(2):356-363. DOI: 10.1039/c7bm00891k

[33] Soeki T, Tamura Y, Shinohara H, Sakabe K, Onose Y, Fukuda N. Serum hepatocyte growth factor predicts ventricular remodeling following myocardial infarction. Circulation Journal. 2002;**66**:1003-1007

[34] Heeschen C, Dimmeler S, Hamm CW, et al. Prognostic significance of angiogenic growth factor serum levels in patients with acute coronary syndromes. Circulation. 2003;**107**(4):524-530. DOI: 10.1161/01/CIR/0000048183.37648.1A

[35] Teplyakov AT, Berezikova EN, Shilov SN, Grakova EV, Torim YY, Efremova AV. i soavt. Patogeneticheskaya i prognosticheskaya znachimost rostovyh faktorov v razvitii hronicheskoj serdechnoj nedostatochnosti. Kardiologiya—Cardiology. 2017;**57**(10):20-28. DOI: 10.18087/cardio.2017.10.10039 (in russ)

[36] Yusuf S, Hawken S, Ounpuu S, et al. Effect of potentially modifiable risk factors associated with myocardial infarction in 52 countries (the INTERHEART study): Case-conrol study. Lancet. 2004;**364**(9438):937-952. DOI: 10.1016/S0140-6736(04)17018-9

[37] Surtees PG, Wainwright NWJ, Luben RN, Wareham NJ, Bingham SA, Khaw K-T. Psychological distress, major depressive disorder, and risk of stroke. Neurology. Mar 2008;**70**(10):788-794. DOI: 10.1212/01.wnl.0000304109.18563.81

[38] Doering LV, Moser DK, Riegel B, et al. Persistent comorbid symptoms of depression and anxiety predict mortality in heart disease. International Journal of Cardiology. 2010;**145**(2):188-192. DOI: 10.1016/j.ijcard.2009.05.025

[39] Versteeg H, Hoogwegt MT, Hansen TB, et al. Depression, not anxiety, is independently associated with 5-year hospitalization and mortality in patients with ischemic heart disease. Journal of Psychosomatic Research. 2013;**75**(6):409-413. DOI: 10.1016/j.jpsychores.2013.10.005

[40] Beach SR, Januzzi JL, Mastromauro CA, Healy BC, Beale EE, Celano CM, Huffman JC. Patient Health Questionnaire-9 score and adverse cardiac outcomes in patients hospitalized for acute cardiac disease. Journal of Psychosomatic Research. 2013 Nov;**75**(5):409-413. DOI: 10.1016/j.jpsychores.2013.08.001. [Epub 2013 Aug 13]

[41] Sotelo JL, Nemeroff CB. Depression as a systemic disease. Personalozed Medicine in Psychiatry. 2017;**1-2**:11-25. DOI: 10.1016/j.pmip.2016.11.002

[42] Stepoe A, Kivimaki M. Stress and cardiovascular disease. Nature Reviews Cardiology. 2012;**9**(6):360-370. DOI: 10.1038/nrcardio.2012.45

[43] Roslavtseva VV, Salmina AB, Prokopenko SV, et al. The role of vascular endothelial growth factor in the regulation of development and functioning of the brain: New target molecules for pharmacotherapy. Biomedicinskaia Chimiia. 2016;**62**(2):124-133. DOI: 10.1809/PBMC20166202124

[44] Elfving B, Buttenschen HN, Foldager L, et al. Depression and BMI influences the serum vascular endothelial growth factor level. International Journal of Neuropsychopharmacology. 2014;**17**(9):1409-1417. DOI: 10.1017/S1461145714000273

[45] Lee BH, Kim YK. Increased plasma VEGF levels in major depressive or manic episodes inpatients with mood disorders. Journal of Affective Disorders. 2012;**136**:181-184. DOI: 10.1016/j.jad.2011.07.021

[46] Kahl KG, Bens S, Ziegler K, et al. Angiogenic factors in patients with current major depressive disorder comorbid with borderline personality disorder. Psychoendocrinology. 2009;**34**(3):353-357. DOI: 10.1016/j.psyneuen.2008.09.016

[47] Takebayashi M, Hashimoto R, Hisaoka K, et al. Plasma levels of vascular endothelial growth factor and fibroblast growth factor 2 in patients with major depressive disorders. Journal of Neural Transmission. 2010;**117**(9):1119-1122. DOI: 10.1007/s00702-010-0452-1

[48] Wallenstein J, Asberg M, Nygen A, et al. Possible biomarkers of chronic stress induced exhaustion—A longitudinal study. PLoS One. 2016;**11**(5):e0153924. DOI: 10.1371/journal.pone.0153924

[49] Segi-Nishida E, Wamer-Schmidt JL, Duman RS. et al, Electroconvulsive seizure and VEGF increase the proliferation of neural stem-like cells in rat hippocampus. Proceedings of the National Academy of Sciences of the United States of America. 2008;**105**(32):11352-11357. DOI: 10.1073/pnas.07108581105

[50] Warner-Schmidt JL. Dumah RS VEGF is an essential mediator of the neurogenic and behavioral actions of antidepressants. Proceedings of the National Academy of Sciences of the United States of America. 2007;**104**(11):4647-4652. DOI: 10.1073/pnas.0610282104

[51] Nikkheslat N, Zunszain PA, Horowitz MA, et al. Insufficient glucocorticoid signaling and elevated inflammation in coronary artery disease patients with comorbid depression. Brain, Behavior, and Immunity. 2015;**48**:8-18. DOI: 10.1016/j.bbi.2015.02.002

[52] Maingrette F, Dussault S, Dhahri W, et al. Psychological stress impairs ischemia-induced neovascularization: Protective effect of fluoxetine. Atherosclerosis. 2015;**241**(2):569-578. DOI: 10.1016/j.atherosclerosis.2016.06.010

[53] Ibanez B, James S, Agewall S, Antunes MJ, Bucciarelli-Ducci C, Bueno H, et al. ESC Scientific Document Group. 2017 ESC Guidelines for the management of acute myocardial infarction in patients presenting with ST-segment elevation: The Task Force for the management of acute myocardial infarction in patients presenting with ST-segment elevation of the European Society of Cardiology (ESC). European Heart Journal. 2018;**39**(2):119-177

[54] Standards of medical care in diabetes 2017: Summary of revisions. Diabetes Care. 2017;**40**:S4-S5